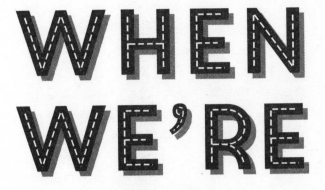

WHEN WE'RE 64

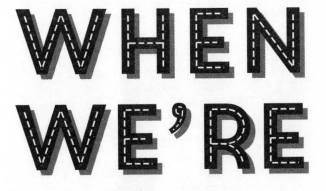

WHEN WE'RE 64

Your Guide to a Great Later Life

LOUISE ANSARI

GREEN TREE
LONDON · OXFORD · NEW YORK · NEW DELHI · SYDNEY

GREEN TREE
Bloomsbury Publishing Plc
50 Bedford Square, London, WC1B 3DP, UK

BLOOMSBURY, GREEN TREE and the Green Tree logo are trademarks of
Bloomsbury Publishing Plc

First published in Great Britain 2019

A catalogue record for this book is available from the British Library

Library of Congress Cataloguing-in-Publication data has been applied for

ISBN: PB: 978-1-4729-6068-9; e-pub: 978-1-4729-6069-6; epdf: 978-1-4729-6070-2

2 4 6 8 10 9 7 5 3 1

Typeset in Minion Pro by Deanta Global Publishing Services, Chennai, India
Printed and bound in Great Britain by CPI Group (UK) Ltd. Croydon, CR0 4YY

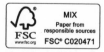

To find out more about our authors and books visit www.bloomsbury.com
and sign up for our newsletters

To all my wonderful colleagues
and to Karen – Ageing Better together!

CONTENTS

INTRODUCTION

This book is going to help you get ready for a major adventure. You are likely to live longer than you think – and I can tell you now, you're not prepared for it. You're not prepared to make it the happiest time of your life. You might have thought about one or two elements – your pension, perhaps, or getting a bit fitter – but there's much more to consider. Not sure where to start? Help is at hand. By the end of this book you'll have the knowledge, tips and pointers to think very differently about the amazing opportunity that a long life can bring…

For those of you who like shortcuts, let me reveal the 10 things that you should do *now* to make sure you prepare to have a great later life. Some of them will surprise you. The rest of this book provides the detail of how to get there. It includes advice on how to change the way you think about the challenges life throws at you, and has lots of practical guidance on subjects ranging from choosing where to live, to how to make sure you'll be financially secure, and much more in between.

So, what are the keys to a great later life?

1. Keep working

You might think older age is all about retirement and a life of leisure. But people want meaning and purpose in their life and, more often than not, work is something that means you can use your brain (or brawn!), connect with others, and obviously it provides a source of income. It's not for everyone – and the work has to be a good, flexible job that suits you – but continuing to work if you can is a really good thing.

2. Stand on one leg

Silly? No. We all know we're supposed to get off the sofa and go jogging – and doing some brisk aerobic activity (75 minutes a week of being breathless, or 150 minutes of moderate activity including fast walking) is a must-do. But one of the keys to a great later life is keeping strength in your muscles and a good ability to balance. Strength and balance are the largely unknown and ignored bits of activity advice for adults. Few people understand their importance, but our strength and balance rapidly decline after the age of 40 and keeping them up could make all the difference between being independent or not when you're older, including reducing the risk of falling.

3. Don't smoke

We all know this one. Or do we? It might be a surprise to learn that 1.3 million people over 60 still smoke in the UK. Smoking causes cancer of the lung, bowel and bladder, and 78,000 people died of smoking-related disease in 2016. Lots of help is available to quit, and vaping is likely to be a good way to wean yourself off cigarettes.

4. Lose weight

What a presumption! I say lose weight because the majority of us are overweight – a shocking 33.3 million people in the UK (that's more than 60 per cent of the population, up from 52 per cent 25 years ago). You might be one of the people who manages to stay at the right point on the body mass index and not have to buy the largest size in the clothes shop, but most of us are not in that happy position. And it does take more conscious effort as we age, as the metabolism slows. Obesity and being overweight leads to Type 2 diabetes, heart disease and an increased risk of several cancers. We know that drinking too much booze can also be harmful, as well as adding calories. So, make the effort and try and lose the extra inches now.

5. Share the love

Making time to help others, from formal volunteering roles like helping at a hospice or fundraising for your favourite charity to just simple things like putting the neighbour's bins out when they're away, has proven benefits for you as well as the people you're helping. Volunteering or contributing in other ways to the community you live in can give the great feeling that you're 'giving back' – but it really is a win-win activity that can add structure and interest to your own life, as well as getting to know new people and learning something new.

6. Be creative

Life isn't all work, of course, however much you might enjoy it (if you do!). Your time in later life will be a great gift, so cultivate yourself, your creativity, your hobbies – the things that make you especially you – now. Some people in retirement do what has been called 'the grab' – trying out a hundred new hobbies and volunteering for everything. If you already know what you enjoy, including learning new things and being creative (bonsai cultivation anyone?), then this will stand you in good stead for a pleasurable use of free time when you're older.

7. Know your place

Are you at home now? Have you thought about whether or not you want to stay in your flat or house as you grow older? If you do, is it going to be right for your needs in terms of space, accessibility and ease of use, and is it in the neighbourhood you want to love in later life? These are serious questions that many people don't think ahead on. Eighty per cent of people aged 65 and over tell us they want to stay in their own home as they grow older, but so many homes aren't fit for purpose. If you want to stay, or move, make that choice a deliberate one, taking into account any future-proofing that your current home needs, or finding the right home in the right place for your needs as you age.

8. Be positive

'One foot in the grave' style grumpiness is out of fashion now we know how a negative attitude to growing old could actually take years off your life. Being downbeat and having a consistently unhappy approach has been associated with a reduction in lifespan of around seven years. I'm not suggesting constant fake smiles, but positivity can help you deal with the slings and arrows of outrageous fortune, as well as keep you healthy physically and mentally from day to day.

9. Save more

If you carry on working, or get back into it if you've left for health reasons or have retired already, this is obviously a good source of income. But saving into a pension, whether it be workplace or private, is absolutely crucial for your financial health as you grow older. Until auto-enrolment (mandatory workplace pensions), 38 per cent of eligible employees had no occupational pension. But with state pension age getting later, and potentially providing you with less income than you'd like or need, saving more is an absolute must in middle age. While the majority of pensioners are in receipt of some state pension, more than ever are supplementing this with private pension income. In 1994, 59 per cent had some private pension benefits. By 2017, this had reached 71 per cent of all pensioners, with only 30 per cent having just the state pension and means-tested benefits to rely on.

10. Happiness is other people

Love, intimacy and good friends are the stuff of life. Sure, we need reasonably good health and enough money to live on, but without sharing our stories and experiences, and without people we could rely on in a crisis, life could be difficult as you get older. Paying attention to your friendships and close relationships in mid-life (both maintaining the ones you've got and connecting with new people) will help enormously as you age. Are most of your friends people at work, for example? Have you thought about how retirement might impact on that?

I'm the Director of Communications at the Centre for Ageing Better, an independent charity. We want a society where everyone enjoys a good later life. I've written this book, with help from my colleagues, to help you start to think differently about all these areas and understand when and how to take action. Even the most organised and informed among you will get new tips on what to do across health, housing, money, relationships and much more, to help prepare you for the great adventure of our fabulously longer lives!

All the resources and websites mentioned in the book are also listed at the back for ease of reference – and while all the info here is correct at the time of writing, many areas (like paying for care) are subject to fast-moving change in policy or legal rights and obligations so check to see if there are updates before taking action.

1

THE 'NEW' ISSUE OF OLD AGE

So. Ageing. What's all the fuss about ageing? Isn't this the oldest, most fundamental human story? We are born, go through childhood, become a teenager, then a young adult with hopes and dreams, pass into middle age and eventually have some (hopefully) serene years of life before we pass away.

No. The story has changed and society (and you?) haven't caught up with that change. Of course, the beginning and the end are still irrefutably birth and death, but it's what's in the middle – and our response to it – that needs a major rethink.

How long do you think you're going to live?

If you're this age now...	You're likely to have this many years ahead...	
	Men	Women
45	41	43
50	35	40
55	30	33
60	25	28
65	21	23
70	17	19
75	13	14

These figures are based on *cohort* life expectancy, which is calculated using observed death rates in your 'cohort' (that is, people born the same year as you). It takes into account actual mortality rates, as well as future changes resulting from likely advances in medicine and technology and improvements in care and treatment.

If we take one of the ways the Office for National Statistics looks at life expectancy, we can see how many years of life have been gained over the last 100 years or so. The modal (or most common) age of death is one of the measurements of how long we might expect to live. This gives us the most common age deaths were registered in any given year. Like other measures of life expectancy, it measures men and women separately. So, in 1900, the most common age of all the women who died that year was 73. By 1975, this had increased to 83, and by 2010, the most common age women died at was 89. For men, the most common age of death in 1900 was 68. In 1975, it was 75, and by 2010, the most common age of men who died was 85. It's increased even further over the last few years. The modal age of death for men between 2015 and 2017 was 86.4.

For decades, life expectancy has been increasing year on year at a fantastic rate. Medical and public health advances, from sanitation to statins, all continue to contribute to reductions in your likelihood of dying before you get old. In 2009, *The Lancet* made the staggering prediction that more than half of British babies born in 2007 will live to the age of 103. In Japan, most children under 10 are expected to live until they are 107. Given that there is better and better treatment and management for long-term conditions, improved cancer survival rates, and better understanding of how we can stay healthy, we are all likely to live longer on average than even these predictions.

But there are worrying signs that increases in life expectancy have now stalled. The slowdown in gains for the number of years you'll live is particularly marked for women. While an amazing 12.9 weeks per year were added to women's lifespans over the period from 2006 to 2011, this reduced dramatically to just 1.2 weeks per year from 2011 to 2016. It's still an increase – but not as large a one as previously experienced. We don't know the causes of this yet, but the slowdown is most marked in people from poorer communities, further exacerbating inequalities in lifespan as well as quality of life.

There are good, personalised 'how long you're going to live' prediction tools on the BBC and the Office for National Statistics websites. It's worth finding out what your predicted lifespan is, so you can spend time planning how to make those extra years fantastic!

Just how many of these 'old' people, who (if you believe the news) are going to crash the economy and bankrupt the NHS, are there? If your definition of old is 50, then that's 24.4 million of us in the UK alone. And there are around as many people aged 60 and over as there are 19 and below. This is accounted for partly by the baby boomer 'bulge' starting in the mid-1950s and finishing in the early 1970s, with more than 14 million babies born by 1972. This group is passing through the years 'like a pig moving through a python' as anthropologist Helen Fisher once put it. Delightful.

This has implications for the future. By 2030 there will be:

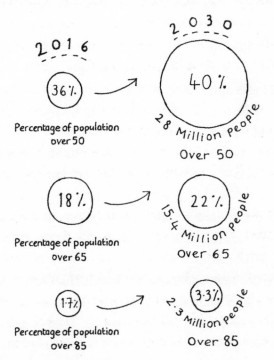

2016
36%
Percentage of population over 50

2030
40%
28 Million people
Over 50

18%
Percentage of population over 65

22%
15.4 Million people
Over 65

1.7%
Percentage of population over 85

3.3%
2.3 Million people
Over 85

But our ageing society isn't just accounted for by the baby boomer generation getting older. As noted above, all of us are living much longer.

And we're not alone in having more years of life. People are living longer everywhere. Global life expectancy is now averaging at 72 years old. An amazing five years have been added to average lifespans globally since the millennium. In the year 2000, average life expectancy was only 50.8 in Africa, and 72.5 in Europe. Within 16 years, Europeans have gained five years, and more than a decade has been added to African life expectancy.

Overall, it's a great achievement and gift that we're living longer. But the average figures hide a picture that's less rosy for some. Today in the UK, the wealthiest 65-year-old men live another 22 years, but the poorest only another 15 years. If you live in Kensington and Chelsea you'll live for longer, and in better health, than if you live in Glasgow. We seem to accept this awful situation, or at least brush it under the carpet – but shouldn't the gift of a longer life be there for all of us?

The quality of life as well as the length of it differs significantly between different groups. People who are poorer financially report being in worse health – they are more likely to have complaints such as depression or poor eyesight and are more likely to suffer from multiple long-term conditions – than people who are better off. Inequalities in how we age can even be seen by how fast people walk. An average person aged 71 in the richest wealth bracket has a walking speed of 0.91 metres per second, compared with 0.75 for someone in the poorest wealth bracket. This matters because it's an indicator not just of how quickly you can get to the shops and back, but of overall health.

As I'll show in the following chapters, there's a lot you can do yourself, whatever your income level, to avoid being in the group who miss out on having a good later life (and it doesn't involve moving to Chelsea!). The health chapter later in this book holds many of the keys – keeping as healthy as you can for as long as you can is at least partly in your control. Having a house that's right for your needs in an area that's 'age-friendly' is something you may be able to change. Staying financially secure is crucially important. And having strong relationships that are good for your mental health will add to your quality of life as you get older.

How old is old age?

After all this talk of demographics, and some thoughts about how many years you might have left, what age do you consider to be the start of being 'old'? 50? 90? ELSA is not just a lovely old-fashioned name but also the acronym for the English Longitudinal Study on Ageing – a fantastic resource that has followed around 10,000 people over the age of 50 for 15 years so far, measuring their attitudes and experience of life as they grow older. According to ELSA, the proportion of people who consider themselves old actually declines with age, from 77 per cent of those in their 50s considering themselves old to 63 per cent of people in their 60s! It's also known from research that people think 'old' is 10 years older than they currently are.

Around the world, there are very different expectations of when youth ends and old age begins. In Britain, most people think youth ends at 35 and old age apparently begins at 59. But technically, and as more of us live past 100, our 50s still seems to be middle age, don't you think? Turkish people are the only other people on the European continent who think we are definitively 'old' in our 50s. Our neighbours in France think 63 is old, and the venerable Greeks define 68 as the start of old age. Have you changed your mind about the age that denotes 'old'? Or are you already enlightened enough to realise that age is more a state of mind than a number on a birthday card?

So there we have it. You have many years ahead. If you're 50 now, you may have another 50 years to go. For some people that thought fills them with dread rather than joy, but let's find a happy medium (though perhaps erring on the 'joy' side) and both imagine and plan for the best that your later life can be, whatever your starting point.

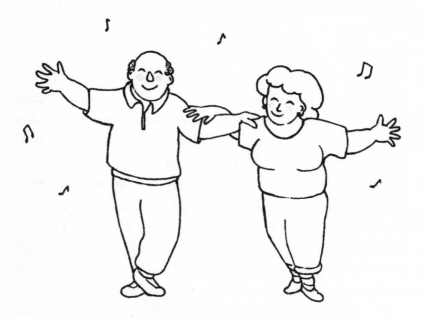

2
HOW ARE YOU AGEING?

There is great diversity among the millions of people over 50 – so frequently lumped together as a homogenous group of 'older people' – but also some distinct groupings. And unlike popular media portrayal, they are not two groups solely comprised of poor, sad, lonely folk or rich, golf-playing socialites. The huge variety of people in later life is an untold story; so, we at the Centre for Ageing Better commissioned research to highlight some of the range of attitudes and ways of life that people in later life experience.

Of course, everyone's different, and how every individual will experience later life is different. But perhaps you can identify yourself, your friends or your family members in some of the groups below?

We asked polling company Ipsos MORI to survey 1,389 older people, making sure the sample was representative of the UK population over 50. From both this and a series of more in-depth studies with a smaller group who completed a diary and gave face-to-face interviews, they were able to give us a snapshot of how people experience life.

They identified and characterised six distinct groups: 'Thriving Boomers', 'Downbeat Boomers', 'Can Do and Connected', 'Worried and Disconnected', the 'Squeezed Middle', and 'Struggling and Alone'. The proportion of people in each group is shown overleaf.

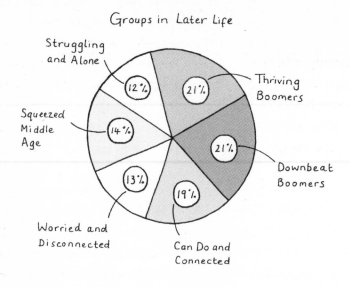

Groups in Later Life

Struggling and Alone — 12%

Thriving Boomers — 21%

Squeezed Middle Age — 14%

Downbeat Boomers — 21%

Worried and Disconnected — 13%

Can Do and Connected — 19%

Thriving Boomers

One of the largest groups identified was the 'Thriving Boomers'. This group is strong in terms of their health, financial stability and social connections. Most had well-paid jobs before retiring and could save to enjoy a high standard of living in later life. Most of this group have assets to fall back on if they need to, usually property. As a result, 91 per cent agreed when asked if they felt they always or almost always had enough money to buy what they needed.

However, it's not just financial independence that means 'Thriving Boomers' are in a comfortable position, but also their relative health in comparison to others their age. Fewer than one-tenth considered themselves to be in fair or poor health, with the overwhelming majority enjoying good health. Although they are largely hale and hearty, this group also identified that if they did experience ill health or a serious problem, they would be able to seek support from friends or a family member.

One important aspect that makes this group different from some of the others is that they largely have a positive mental attitude towards their lives and experiences. When asked to rate their happiness the day before the survey, thriving boomers were significantly more likely to rate their happiness highly (around a 9 or 10 out of 10) than people in other groups. They also feel more in control of their lives, and are more likely to go to cultural events, like visiting a museum. This group also feel they can contribute to their own health, usually exercising regularly and following a healthy diet.

As well as scoring highly on wellbeing, people in this group value social relationships and interaction much more strongly than other groups. In valuing relationships with people in different age groups, such as grandchildren, they forge strong social connections with lots of people, meaning perhaps they're less likely to feel like a burden if they fell ill or needed help.

Downbeat Boomers

People say money can't buy you happiness, and it seems to be true. The most financially secure of all the groups were dubbed the 'Downbeat Boomers'. Nearly all members of this group own their own home, and almost 8 in 10 have paid off their mortgage, but people in this category did not report feeling happy. Even though they were objectively wealthier than most, nearly a third said they didn't always have sufficient funds to cover everything they wanted.

Their negative attitude towards later life means that, instead of thriving, 'Downbeat Boomers' are pessimistic about the future and often regretful about the past and perceived missed opportunities. Slightly more than 2 in 10 of all those questioned for the survey were classed as 'Downbeat Boomers', the most typical profile being that of someone in their 60s and in a relationship.

Given that they are largely well off and in relative good health, this section of the over-50s population reports lower wellbeing scores than you'd expect. About 60 per cent of this group is in good health, but this didn't mean that they considered themselves happy or fortunate. When asked to rate how happy they had been the day before, 60 per cent of this group gave scores lower than 9, with most giving scores of just 'fair' or worse, or less than 8 out of 10.

So, although financial stability is one of the key aspects identified as being important in later life, it's clearly not everything. Even though things may seem to be going well for the 'Downbeat Boomers', their happiness scores lag behind the other groups. Personality, outlook and disposition play a hugely significant role in the way that people view their later life and this group see their lives in a mostly pessimistic way. We'll return to the subject of attitudes to old age and how important they are in a later chapter.

Can Do and Connected

In contrast to the downbeat boomers, the 'Can Do and Connected' group show the great impact a positive attitude towards later life can have. Nearly 20 per cent of people in the study fell into this category. Although facing more challenges, this group adopt a more optimistic, 'can do' attitude towards their lives and the future, mostly because of how much they enjoy social interactions and relationships.

Just over a third of this group describe their health as 'fair' or 'poor', and so are one of the least healthy groups identified. These respondents were the oldest in the study, the majority being widowed women in their 70s and 80s. But despite their ill health, they are confident they would be able to draw on close relationships and friendships for support if they needed to and feel that they are fortunate. The fact that this group has a large support network means that they feel more comfortable asking for help, and they're likely to ask for it, feeling that they had helped others in the past.

As well as poor physical health, this group isn't particularly wealthy. Either because of ill health or childcare, most people who fall under this category have either not worked or have been in and out of employment for most of their lives. Consequently, they have little saved for their future, and 35 per cent felt they didn't have enough money for their needs in their later lives.

Despite these challenges, almost half of this group said they were extremely happy. The key to contentment for this group of over-50s is their positivity and making connections and forming relationships to help them through later life.

Worried and Disconnected

While the 'Can Do and Connected' group showed the benefits of developing and keeping strong social connections, 13 per cent of the 'Worried and Disconnected' group could not identify someone they would be able to rely on in an emergency. Instead of feeling able to ask for help, 'Worried and Disconnected' people are anxious about becoming or being a burden. Generally, they're over 70, retired and in poor health. This group have difficulty making connections with new people, and don't feel comfortable reaching out to friends or family for support.

The 'Worried and Disconnected' often lack meaningful human interactions and have weak social relationships. Relationships that help others to overcome health problems and financial strain just don't exist here. On top of this, a significant proportion of this group are in poor health – so their lack of a support system is a problem.

The disconnect between this group of over-50s and wider society resulted in nearly one in six reporting happiness scores between 0 and 5, on the very lowest end of the scale.

Some of this group are older, widowed women. They imagined that their husbands would take care of the financial planning in their later years, as they had always done. Unused to managing finances, these women do not want to become a burden to family and friends, but do not feel comfortable asking for help.

Squeezed Middle

As the title suggests, this group is still in mid-life. Often, they're still working. But, despite earning a good wage, this group feels financially pressed. This is because of high outgoings and multiple demands on their time and money. With looking after parents and financially dependent children added to their expenses, they've not got much left over to save for retirement.

Despite knowing that later life is approaching, people in the 'Squeezed Middle' find themselves unable to properly prepare, given the demands of the present. In terms of finance and time, many in this category are stretched. Not only that, they feel they don't have enough space in their home. This, and other anxieties rooted in their everyday lives, means that a third feel unhappy. This 'squeezed' feeling leaves little room for thoughts about the distant or even near future.

In comparison to 'Thriving Boomers', often 20 years their senior, this group is in worse health, and nearly half stated that they often or very often did not have enough funds to cover expenses. They usually rejected the idea of asking for help, and their personal experience of caring for, or seeking care for, their parents put them in something of a state of denial – they avoid making provision for their own later life or even thinking much about it.

With so little time and money, this group struggle to find time for themselves, or make meaningful relationships they would be able to count on in their later years. More than 10 per cent thought that they would have no-one to call on in an emergency for support.

Struggling and Alone

The group that measures the worst on all outcomes were named 'Struggling and Alone'. A third of those who fall into this group find themselves frequently or always short of money. Unlike the other sections, people in this group do not fall into approximate age brackets but cover a range of ages. Many people in this group live alone and experience depression.

More than a third of people questioned in this group categorised their health as poor, and many had taken time out of their careers before retiring due to illness. Many had been ill or disabled for many years, and so hadn't been able to save for a good later life. An inconsistent or infrequent working life also meant that this group had made fewer lasting social connections that they could rely on. Nearly a quarter of 'Struggling and Alone' people didn't feel they would have someone to rely on in an emergency – the lowest percentage of any of the respondent groups.

Poor health, poor financial prospects and few social connections meant that this group often found itself isolated and unhappy. Nearly three-quarters described their happiness the day before they were questioned as falling somewhere between 0 and 5 out of 10.

****

So, what does all this mean for you? If you could identify yourself more or less in one of the 'happier' groups like 'Thriving Boomer' or 'Can do and Connected', great! If you perhaps related more to 'Worried and Disconnected' or 'Squeezed Middle', don't despair, there is support you can access and things you can do to change your circumstances. In further analysis, we found some movement between these groups over time – but it tended to mostly be movement towards a less happy, financially stable life. This is something for everyone to guard against. Whether life gets better or not as we grow old depends on building and maintaining your health, your financial security, your relationships, and your positive attitude to ageing, as well as preparing for expected and unexpected life events.

How all these changes affect you will obviously be different for everyone, but planning ahead and taking action now across all these areas will mean you have more control over how changes (like retirement or choosing to work for longer) and health events (like a diagnosis of a long-term condition) impact on you. You might not relate to any of these segments – or you might find something of your situation in bits of all of them. You might recognise them as describing the way a colleague, friend or family member sees life. Categorisation can over-simplify the great diversity and uniqueness of each and every one of us, but this doesn't deny that having the best possible later life will take some dedication and action from everyone...

3

ARE YOU AN OLD AGE AGEIST?

What is ageism? How does our perception of age affect how we think about our later lives, and how is that perception affected by the media, advertising, and other people's attitudes?

The term ageism is widely thought to have been coined by Robert Butler, an American gerontologist, in the late 1960s. Butler's two bestselling books, *Why Survive? Being Old in America* and *Love and Sex after 60*, gave name to a kind of discrimination that many were familiar with and was widely accepted. There are a lot of expressions of ageism in the world – from demeaning terms for older people, to discrimination in employment, or in services like healthcare. And as well as these external expressions of negativity about growing older, we can be ageist about ourselves. If we have a negative attitude or deep distaste, or even revulsion, about old age, we are feeling negative about something that we will all – unless we die young – experience. This 'internalised' ageism impacts on the way we behave as we grow older. Perhaps we loathe or are at best unhappy with the likelihood of getting older, sicker, lonelier and ultimately dying. Is it our fear of death that leads us to fear ageing? In 1989, Butler said we need to re-imagine how we see old age, and what we see as valuable in longer lives. That's still true today.

So how does ageism manifest itself? Once you start looking for it, you see it everywhere, from people jovially writing themselves off ('I'm over the hill now'), to a reinforcement in media articles of older age being a time of stupidity and worthlessness. Can you spot which of these are genuine headlines?

Pensioner 'who doesn't like men' drives mobility scooter into one police officer and hits another with bottle

Robot CATS to be used to help elderly people with tasks and reminders

Forgetful elderly couple offer £100 reward if someone can find their car they lost FOUR days ago

Pensioner dies after swallowing his wedding ring without knowing it

Paranoid granny spends £4,000 defending her home against wi-fi signals

Sex robots could be used by the elderly to help them overcome anxiety and erectile dysfunction

Yes, you guessed it – they're all true. (I'm intrigued about the robot cats idea!) Ageism is everywhere: on our TV screens, in the cinema and on the radio, and in this regard, it particularly seems to affect women. In 2013, only 26 of the 481 news presenters over 50 across all major UK networks were women. More often than not, men are allowed to age on our screens, while middle-aged and older women get replaced with younger versions. This also happens on the big screen, of course. Maggie Gyllenhaal revealed a few years ago that she'd been dismissed as being too old – at the age of 37 – for the role of love interest to a 55-year-old man. And in contrast, Denzel Washington, who's 63, had never had an onscreen romance with a woman older than 35 until the film of the play 'Fences'.

One of the most noticeable ways that ageism is expressed is, of course, in language – in the names and terms that some people use to describe people in later life. Codger, fogey, biddy, crone, OAP, little old lady, geriatric. Not exactly a life-affirming picture – more the description of a narrow-minded, incapable, foolish or cantankerous person. I think we're probably becoming a bit more sensitive in not using terms like this (particularly the more of us there are in later life!) – but there are some others that annoyingly seem to stick around. Every now and again, for example, I get called 'young lady', normally by a shopkeeper mentally stuck in the 1980s. I know it's meant almost as a jokey compliment, but it does make me raise an eyebrow. I fear that as I get older, I will become more and more subject to, 'What can I get for you, young lady?' daftness. We haven't yet found a set of words that people are happy with to describe ageing. The really hard word is the word 'old' itself. As I noted in Chapter Two, most of us don't ever use that word to describe ourselves, whatever our age. We think people about 10 years older than us are 'old'. What are the alternatives? Vintage? Distinguished? Mature?! Ageism in the media, broader culture, and in the very language we speak does have an insidious and negative impact on how we think about ageing.

Apart from affecting our image of ourselves, ageism also has a pernicious impact on other major aspects of our lives. According to ELSA, 60 per cent of people over 50 don't think that older people get enough respect in society. People over 50 report high levels of ageism in recruitment to jobs, promotions and whether or not they're offered training at work. We recently commissioned a YouGov poll and found that one in five over-50s believe they've been turned down for a job because of their age. And although a third thought they received fewer training opportunities and chances for progression than younger workers, only 1 per cent had complained about ageism in their workplace. In the health service, ageism can affect the way healthcare professionals treat people – and this can even mean they are not considered worthy of treatment. At the most extreme and horrific end, ageism has led to high-profile cases of doctors putting an end to the life of people over 60. Even the son of one of Harold Shipman's victims said, 'It is murder, but I would like to think of it as euthanasia'.

Are you experiencing ageism?

Let's have a quick check-in about how *you* feel about 'old age'. Do you think it will be a depressing, lonely time of your life? What do you think will happen in terms of your health and physical independence? Some might say 'my identity is not defined by how old I am', or be more positive and expect that their experience will make them more valued. Some will be more accepting of who they are as the years pass. Does this reflection show you're thinking about ageing positively, or with some sadness and regret?

There is some good news. According to ELSA, only one in 10 people think that their age prevents them from doing what they want. And while it's a slim-ish majority, 60 per cent of people have viewed getting older as a positive experience. Getting that to 100 per cent might be unrealistic, but let's start with ourselves…

Dr Hannah Swift is a research fellow at the University of Kent and has a deeper explanation of why we think about age the way we do, and how 'internalised ageism' impacts on us:

'When we're younger, we learn stereotypes and traits about people at different ages. The stereotypes aren't all bad – they can be positive as well as negative. When I ask children to draw pictures of older people, they draw people with walking sticks, but also describe older people as warm and friendly, if not competent or able to get around!

'Those stereotypes you learnt when you were young about older people? You start applying them to yourself. A recognised stereotype, for example, is "I'm too old for that," and you will start applying that at various ages. When you're 30, for example, you might say "I'm too old to go clubbing now". When you're 70 you might say, "I'm too old to travel the world now". It's a way of modifying our behaviour, not according to our actual ability (because of course we can go clubbing or travelling at any age we want), but according to stereotypes of age. Of course, we should try and break these frames of thinking – some need revising more than others, like "I'm too old to work".

'So how can we break these stereotypes that are so embedded in our psyche? It's a bit to do with awareness about your own attitudes to ageing and how you feel about getting older yourself. If you feel negative about ageing, then that's likely to be a self-fulfilling prophesy. But of course, lots of this negativity or denial is absorbed by us from cues in society, and this is particularly true for women who are surrounded by stereotypes about what you should look like at every age. It's a market of creams, hair dyes, magic solutions and impossible images to make us resist ageing. Be accepting of who you really are, and don't limit what you can do "because of your age", or your potential to do more, or do things differently in the future. I'd also advise friendships with people in different age groups. If you have really good friends who are much older or younger, that will break some of the stereotypes!'

Ageism kills

So, by now we've got a rough idea of how long we might live. Factors like whether you smoke or not, how much you drink and what you eat, and whether or not you do enough exercise will have a huge impact on your longevity (I'll talk much more about this in Chapter Six on health). And we're starting to understand that the way you think can also add or subtract years from your life. As well as the ageism prevalent in society, our own attitudes to life and growing older – the very way *we think* – could impact on not just the quality of life we have as we age, but the *actual number of years we live.* Yes – the way you think might shorten or lengthen your life. It's a pretty mind-blowing idea that you could actually think yourself a longer life. Now this is only one study, carried out by Professor Becca Levy from Yale University in 2002, but it showed that people who are positive about later life live a staggering 7.5 years more than those who are negative about their own ageing.

How does this work? I spoke to Guy Robertson, an expert in attitudes towards ageing, who runs a consultancy called Positive Ageing Associates. He explained to me that being optimistic and having a positive take on life in general (about the small things as well as big events) leads to you not just being happier, but healthier – which leads to the extra years. I'm a fairly optimistic soul, but I pretended to be a grumpy middle-aged woman (it wasn't hard) so that Guy could advise me directly on what to do.

'You can change. Some people are more optimistic, or more pessimistic, but these are not character traits written on tablets of stone. There is the possibility to change the way you think. It all comes down to being aware of your thought patterns. I'll tell you why that's important.

'Ask people what creates a feeling, and they will say, "I feel this way because this particular thing has happened to me". This is not true. There's an intermediate step – after the event happens, there's a thought about the event, an interpretation, a set of assumptions. This is what causes the feeling, not the event itself.

'If something happens to a pessimistic person – say they lose their wallet, for example – a downbeat person will think, "Oh God, what a disaster. It's my fault. This sort of thing always happens to me. My whole life is pretty s**t in fact. This is the straw that broke the camel's back."

'But someone who has a more optimistic outlook might say, "Bugger. That's a problem. I might have dropped it, or someone might have picked my pocket. It's not necessarily my fault. It's a drag, but I know what to do. I can cancel my bank cards and borrow ten quid off John at work. It won't stop me enjoying my weekend."

'If you try and become more aware of your thought responses to events, you can slowly train yourself to respond more positively – this will have a profound effect on your emotional wellbeing. So, we have established that thoughts lead to feelings, not events in themselves. And if you feel positive, you are more likely to behave in a positive and self-protecting way. It's almost certain you'll have a poorer later life if you behave in a negative way and have a downer on yourself because negative attitudes can lead to self-limiting ideas. Negative attitudes are the ones that make people say, "I'm 70 now so I shouldn't bother the doctor about the pain in my back. It's just going to be normal for someone my age. I'll just suffer in silence."

'The way we think about ageing has a huge impact on outcomes for us – how likely we are to get ill, how fast we will recover from illness and how fully, how our memory performs, and even our ability to do simple activities of daily life like getting out of a chair. Negative attitudes have such a severe impact that they could literally kill you.'

This all made sense. But in my pessimistic persona I was feeling quite dubious – it sounds pretty difficult to change the way you think.

'Yes, of course. This can't happen overnight. Like physical exercise, you should start slowly, and you have to put the work in. Begin to be aware of the way you think and try and respond differently next time something bad happens or you have a negative thought about the future. And by the way, I'm not suggesting we should be relentlessly positive about everything. Negative feelings are important in life. This isn't about eradicating sadness. It's about checking and correcting a tendency to be our own worst enemy. Shift yourself a little bit along the scale to be a bit more optimistic, not a zealot of positivity.'

Guy's advice applies to other areas of change – be conscious about what you want to change and self-aware when it comes to thought patterns and the behaviour that leads to. Take small steps to retrain your brain, starting slowly and forgiving yourself for lapses. We'll return to how to help change for the better if you feel you need or want to as we go through the book.

Millennial myths

Of course, not all ageism is directed at older people. 'Millennials' –
people born between the early 1980s and late 1990s – get a bad rep
sometimes. Polling company Ipsos MORI looked at the evidence and
busted some myths about this group of people, who make up around a
quarter of the population.

- They're not 'lazier' than other generations, nor do they change jobs
  more than people at other ages.
- They don't feel deep resentment towards baby boomers. When asked
  to describe this older age group, in the MORI study they used words
  including 'respectful', 'work-centric', 'community-oriented', 'well-
  educated' and 'ethical'.
- It is true that they're not able to afford homes in the way that the
  previous generation were, and fewer are getting married and having
  children at a young age.

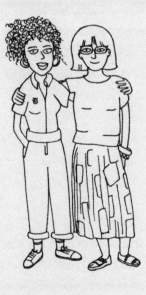

****

So, we've looked at some of the forces ranged against us as we grow older. These include ageism in society and attitudes to older people that can have serious effects like pushing people out of the job market (there's more on this and what to do about it in Chapter Five on work later). We have learnt that thinking positively about ageing can potentially help us live longer and that self-directed ageism means that we can be our own worst enemy sometimes. Let's take a few small steps. If you start thinking negatively about your prospects (in working, being active, having adventures), challenge yourself to think a bit differently. If you're positive about ageing and can see that others aren't, give them a pep talk (and lend them this book after you've finished it!). If you're angry about ageism, campaign against it! Write to the papers or advertisers to blast any stereotypes of ageing you see. Make change happen in your local area (perhaps by getting involved with the Age-Friendly Cities and Communities movement that I talk about in Chapter Seven on where you'll live).

And next time you're buying a birthday card for a friend, maybe choose a different slogan than those opposite…

And yes – you guessed it – the wording is all based on real cards.

40

is still young !

If you're...

a tortoise

or

an oak tree

HAPPY 50th

Though she fought it with every fibre of her being, on her **50th** she let nature take its course and became the proud owner of a tartan shopping bag on wheels

---

60

Too **Old** for a Midlife Crisis

Too **young** for velcro shoes

HAPPY 70TH BIRTHDAY !

He hadn't managed to make a call on his smartphone , but he did have **17** photos of his left ear !

4

FUNDING IT

Money. That's what I want. That's what we all want. Lots of lovely money to go on cruises, go to the theatre, and watch the great rock stars from our youth who have come out of retirement again for another farewell tour. We need money to travel the world, stock our gardens and treat our partners to dinner at Michelin-starred restaurants. We need a LOT of money to live the fantasy retirement lifestyle. Or do we? Most people I know say that they don't want to be rich, they just want to feel financially secure. They don't hanker after the hot tickets or designer fashion. They just want to be able to pay the rent or mortgage (or pay the mortgage off), to be able to cover food and bills, and have some extra money to pursue hobbies. Importantly, people also want to have enough money as they grow older for unexpected events, and to pay for care if necessary. In fact, the percentage of people who think masses more money will make them happy goes down with every age bracket – from 55 per cent of 18–24-year-olds to only 7 per cent of over 75s. People don't want millions; they want enough.

But working out how much is enough, and how to make sure you have it, is a different kettle of fish. This is particularly true for those of us who are not guaranteed large final salary workplace pensions, and of course no-one gets a significant amount of income from a state pension. The bottom line is that we all need to take a long hard look at our finances and try and make some predictions about what we'll need every year for the rest of our life. Then we need to figure out what that might mean for the number of years we

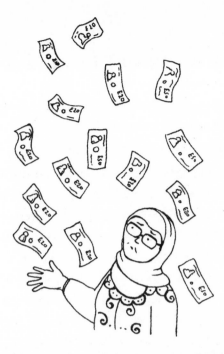

need to work, how much we need to save into pensions and other savings products like ISAs, and what other sources of income could be. Some of us might be able to get benefits to help top up income. And many of us will need to consider how much we may need to contribute to the cost of our care. This chapter gives advice on all of these areas, but I should say that this is a fast-moving area of policy change. How much tax we will need to pay, how care is funded (including by self-funding, and selling housing assets), and how much state pension and other benefits we'll receive and when, are all likely to change significantly over the next few decades, even if this is a politically sensitive area and increasing tax or paying for care isn't usually a vote winner. But while this context is really important, most of us have a fair amount of control over our finances and can make choices in middle age that should lead us to having financial security in later life – the 'just enough' amount of money that's right for each of us.

Working longer

This is the moment of dread for many people. The rough calculations have been done and the penny drops about the need for almost everyone to work longer than they might have imagined; certainly to state pension age and probably beyond, primarily for financial reasons. We will need income to keep paying bills, and for food and housing costs, and we'll need to keep paying into pensions because we haven't got enough in the pots yet. The next chapter covers work at length, and how to help frame it differently for yourself. Because sometimes people do miss the fundamentals of work: if you have the choice about where to work, and for how long, you are far less likely to 'dread' work. This is especially true if it's good work that makes you feel like you're making a contribution, is sociable, or deepens your knowledge. But the money it generates and your ability to save is crucial for you to be able to enjoy your later life.

The big P...

Everyone's talking about pensions these days. It might be my age, but everywhere I turn I'm urged to put more into a private pension, told I have been auto-enrolled into a work pension anyway, and to top it all, hear that I'll be getting the state pension later than I thought. Then I see stories about reckless 60-somethings who use their new pension freedoms to cash it all in and buy a Ferrari, ignoring people who tell them, 'the Ferrari won't pay your gas bill in 20 years' time'. Or I read an article that says I need to have a pension pot value of half a million quid in order to get an income of £25,000 a year – and this seems a bit confusing and a little bit frightening, so I turn the page quickly.

This is not unusual. Plenty of people find the intricacies of pensions difficult to get to grips with. And if we're talking about more people needing help with their pension options, those who are most at risk of shortfalls, but who feel they know the least about pensions, largely seem to be women. An Office for National Statistics survey on attitudes towards pensions found that, in every age bracket below state pension age, men were 15 per cent more confident that they knew enough to make financial decisions about their later life. In the over-65s category, men were 18 per cent more likely to feel like they knew enough about pensions to cope. If you've taken a long time out of paid work to raise children or care for a relative, you might be very unsure that you understand how it all works.

But perhaps you take it for granted that you'll get a pension – and that it will be more or less enough. Maybe you've got a combination of the state pension and one or more employer pensions. This section aims to shine a clear light on the perplexing world of pensions and point you to where to get further advice that suits your specific situation.

Pensions are a problem in Britain, both for the state and for many individuals.

- In 2014, only 36 per cent of women aged 65 to 69 were able to claim the full state pension. This is because you need to have made at least 10 years of National Insurance contributions to receive a state pension at all, and you need 35 or more years to qualify for the full entitlement. This can mean women who take time off work to have children and don't claim child benefit or allowances for caring for loved ones miss out. There are 1.9 million pensioners, many of them single women, classed as living in poverty, living on less than 60 per cent of the median income after housing costs.
- People underestimate how much they'll need for retirement by a significant amount. On average, people think they'll need £124,000, in addition to the state pension, in their pension pots to have a retirement income of £25,000 a year. In reality, you'd need about £315,000 to

achieve this amount of income. More than half of those under 35 thought they'd need less than £100,000.

- In 2006, 38 per cent of eligible employees had no occupational pension. But there is some good news – as auto-enrolment has been rolled out, more people are contributing to workplace pensions. By 2016, only 22 per cent of those eligible had no occupational pension. As all eligible workers had to be auto-enrolled by February of 2018, this is likely to have dropped even further.

- When the modern state pension was introduced in 1948, a 65-year-old could expect to spend 13.5 years in receipt of it – 23 per cent of their adult life. This has been increasing ever since. In 2017, a 65-year-old could expect to live for another 22.8 years, or 33.6 per cent of their adult life.

Increasing the state pension age

The number of people over state pension age in the UK is expected to grow by a third between 2017 and 2042, from 12.4 million in 2017 to 16.9 million in 2042. In response to this, the Government commissioned eminent business and employment expert Sir John Cridland to carry out a review of the state pension age in 2016.

Looking both at the affordability of the pension bill, public finances overall, the likely rise in the amount paid out with increasing longevity, and other factors such as people working for longer, he recommended increasing the state pension age from 66 to 68. The Government took on these recommendations and proposed a timetable for implementation. The state pension age will increase to age 68 in stages (although it's not yet known exactly how) between 2037 and 2039 – affecting everyone born on or after 6 April 1970.

There will be more pension reviews in the future, so keep abreast of changes. Look at the website Gov.uk for all the latest on pension ages and entitlements.

The hidden scandal of lower pensions for women

Women face specific challenges when it comes to pensions. The problem lies in a combination of factors: women are much more likely to spend time out of the labour market, leave work earlier, and are paid less than men when they're working. Analysis by Citizens Advice has found that they are significantly less likely to meet the income threshold requirement of £10,000 to trigger auto-enrolment into workplace pensions. They estimate that 72,000 women are missing out on auto-enrolment because their income is spread over several jobs, with no single job meeting the threshold. As well as this, they're likely to have more years of retirement they need to fund. In 2017, women on average received £126.45 state pension per week, compared to £153.99 for men. Women born in the 1950s who will have to work for longer due to changes in the pension age are likely to be particularly short-changed. The WASPI (Women Against State Pension Inequality) campaign says the changes to increase women's pension age to 66 did not give people enough notice and were made faster than promised, leaving many to rapidly have to change their retirement plans.

Pension essentials

I won't be able to explore every detail on pensions in this chapter – there are whole books dealing with the topic – but here are a few key points to remember:

- Work out what income you think you'll need when you retire. You need to plan early and think about your likely future needs.
- Don't depend just on the state pension to provide your income in retirement – if you are able to put money into work or private pension schemes, do so!
- Even if you are auto-enrolled into a workplace pension, chances are that you're still not putting enough by, so think about ways to increase

your pension savings. If you own your own home, the idea that 'my home is my pension' is a very risky fall-back – we can't predict what's going to happen to the housing market in the future or what the value of your home will be; or how much of your fixed assets you might need to use to pay for care.

And to get more detailed advice, I interviewed Michelle Cracknell, who is the Chief Executive of the Pensions Advisory Service. She explained with crystal clarity how to prepare, and avoid pension pitfalls…

Michelle – first a very basic question: what is a pension?!

'The strict definition of a **pension** is an income paid to you after you have finished work. In practice, the word pension is used to describe a **pension scheme** where you are a member, building up an entitlement to an income in your retirement, and it is also used to describe a **pension pot** where you and possibly your employer are paying in contributions that are invested until you draw an income from it in your retirement.'

What are the different types of pensions?

'Most people have two types of pension; the state pension and private pensions. In private pensions, you may be in a:

- **defined benefit pension scheme** – where you will get an income at retirement based on your years of service and your earnings. Most of these types of scheme have been closed down so you are unlikely to be invited to join one unless you work in some public sector organisations.
- **defined contribution pension scheme** – which is a pension pot where you, and probably your employer, are paying in contributions that are invested until you draw an income from it in your retirement. If you start work with an employer, you will

probably be automatically enrolled into one of these types of workplace pension schemes.'

How much pension will I need when I stop working?

'This is a really good question but there is not one simple answer. Your income in retirement will typically come from your state pension, pensions from your various employments and any other savings that you might have. The amount of pension you will need when you stop working will depend on a number of factors including:

- Your outgoings in retirement;
- Your expectations about what you intend to do in retirement, which are often age related;
- Your health, which will affect how long you may live and any care you may need.'

Will I be able to rely on the state pension?

'The full entitlement of state pension was £164.35 per week in 2017/18 if you have paid or received credits for 35 years of national insurance. For most people, this is barely enough to cover their essential expenses, so they need a private pension and other savings to top up income in retirement.'

In fact, the UK has one of the worst net 'replacement rates' in the 36 OECD (Organisation for Economic Cooperation and Development) countries. This measures what percentage of previous income most people can expect in their retirement. In most OECD countries, the average retiree will have about 63 per cent of their previous salary to live on. In the UK, a person earning an average wage only has about 29 per cent of that income in their retirement if they are relying on the state pension alone.

How much do I need to save or put into pension plans?

'The good news is that if you are employed, you will have been automatically enrolled into your employer's workplace scheme (unless you earn less than £10,000 or are self-employed). If your employer is paying the minimum total contribution, they will be paying 2 per cent of your qualifying earnings and you will be paying 3 per cent. From April 2019, both yours and your employer's contributions will increase. Even better news is that if you pay income tax, you'll get tax relief on your contributions so a contribution of £100 will only cost you £80 and it will be topped up by £20 from the Government.

'Again, for most people, putting in the minimum total contribution into a pension will not provide a big enough pot to provide sufficient income in your retirement. A rule of thumb is that your pension contribution should be half your age when you start putting money into a pension; for example, if you first start a pension at 24, the total contributions going into your pension while you are working should be 12% of your earnings. In practice, people's contributions are more haphazard throughout their working life as the priorities for their money change. Here are some tips:

- If your employer offers matching contributions, you should try to take advantage of them; for example, if for every 1 per cent you contribute, your employer will match up to a maximum employer contribution of 10 per cent, try and contribute as high a percentage as you can.
- If your employer offers salary sacrifice, and you earn above the average earnings, this is a very tax efficient way to make pension contributions as you pay lower National Insurance. Salary sacrifice involves giving up part of your salary in return for benefits promised by your employer – in this case, pension contributions.
- If you have fluctuating earnings, make pension contributions in the years that you are paying higher rate tax as you get tax relief at your highest marginal rate, so it will cost you less.

- There are tools available on most providers' websites that can help you work out how much you should be contributing.'

I've heard about new pension freedoms – that you can cash in pots you have built up. What are the pros and cons of doing this?

'If you have a defined contribution pension pot, from the age of 55, you can start taking your benefits. There are a number of options such as:

1. Using the pot to buy a guaranteed income that will be paid for the rest of your life (known as an annuity).
2. Drawing an income down from the pot.
3. Cashing in the whole pot.
4. A combination of these options.

'Before deciding, you should take guidance from the Government service, Pension Wise, which will describe each of the options and the pros and cons of each. Further details are available at the Pensions Advisory Service website, though be aware that this service, the Money Advice Service and Pensions Wise are all merging into one single financial advice body, so Gov.uk will give you an up-to-date source of information.

'Remember, the earlier you access your pension, the less it will be worth. If you decide to cash in one or more of your pension pots, you will have to pay tax on the money, and this would also affect any means-tested benefits you might apply for in the future. Twenty-five per cent of the pot is paid tax free with the rest of the pot value added to your other income to calculate the tax payable. It could be better to draw your pot over a number of tax years to reduce the tax.

'If you decide to cash in one or more of your pension pots, you need to have other pensions to live on in your retirement. You will also have a lower annual allowance, which is the amount that you can carry on contributing into your pension that qualifies for tax relief.'

My pension's my house – I'll just release equity from it, so I'm not that worried – should I think differently?

'This is a very risky strategy. As with all investments, you should probably have a number of different types of investments rather than relying on your house to provide you with an income in retirement. Equity release is an option to release some money from your house, for example to cover the cost of long-term care in your later life, but you should get independent advice, so you fully understand how it works. Recently, Age UK have released an information sheet about equity release to help you understand any possible risks and benefits. You can find this, and a lot more, on their website.'

What are the other options for income in later life, apart from continuing to work?

'People are living longer and hence many people are working later in life. When you do stop working, you may have a state pension, pensions from your various employments and other savings that you have.

'Here are some tips to make sure that you have sufficient income in retirement:

- Make sure that you have paid or received credits for 35 years of National Insurance to get a full state pension. If you haven't, you may wish to pay voluntary National Insurance Contributions. It is possible to do this in a number of cases, including if you're not working and not claiming benefits. It's usually only possible to fill in gaps from the last six tax years.
- Check that you know about all of the pensions that you have built up throughout your working life. If you think you have "lost" a pension, the Pensions Advisory Service can help you trace it.
- Make sure that you are making the most of any pension scheme that your employer offers.

- Think about other tax efficient savings such as Individual Savings Accounts (ISAs), which have tax benefits and can offer better rates of interest if you invest in a Cash ISA.

'This may all seem very complicated. There is a public service, The Pensions Advisory Service, that will answer any question that you have on pensions by providing you with personalised guidance. Give them a call!'

Millionaire = short of bread?

While we've looked largely at the need to save more and pension shortfalls, the very well-off among us face a tax charge on saving *too much*. The lifetime allowance of your pension pot in 2018/19 was just over £1 million. This is the value of all pensions you have, including those promised to you in defined benefit pension schemes. It doesn't include state pension. Once you reach this maximum allowance for payouts, you'll be taxed more when you receive them – this would kick in if your retirement income is over £51,500 a year under current regulations, with no separate lump sums. This is a complex and fast-moving area of change, so study the official advice and tax implications of pension savings and drawdowns if you're in this lucky position!

When is my state pension age?

State pension age for women
If you were born **before 6 April 1950**, your state pension age is 60.

If you were born **on or after 6 April 1950 but before 6 December 1953**, your state pension age will be somewhere between 60 and 65, depending on your date of birth.

If you were born **on or after 6 December 1953 but before 6 April 1978**, your state pension age will be somewhere between 65 and 68, depending on your date of birth.

If you were born **on or after 6 April 1978**, your state pension age will be 68.

State pension age for men
If you were born **before 6 December 1953**, your state pension age is 65.

If you were born **on or after 6 December 1953 but before 6 April 1978**, your state pension age will be somewhere between 65 and 68, depending on your date of birth.

If you were born on or **after 6 April 1978**, your state pension age will be 68.

Gov.uk has up-to-date information on your state pension age, and you can also see if and where you have gaps in contributions to national insurance. The site also has a calculator, which will tell you your exact pension age.

Saving enough *now*

It's easy to sail through life not thinking too much about pensions, particularly if you're automatically enrolled into a workplace scheme. I talked to Rachael, 32, who changed her pension contribution after learning more about the impact of not saving enough.

'I hadn't thought much about pensions – I wasn't in a full-time role until I moved to London when I was 27, then got auto-enrolled into a teacher's pension scheme. I had no idea what was going into it or what it meant. There was a set percentage I think I put in and the employer did as well, but I didn't increase it even though there was the option. Then I got a new job and a couple of years in they put on a presentation about pensions for staff, and at the same time, coincidentally, I received a 3 per cent cost of living raise in my salary.

Just listening to someone talk about the importance of it and thinking about it a bit more prompted me to add a further 2 per cent of my salary to the scheme. I didn't understand everything in the presentation, but it made me think about what lifestyle I want when I'm older. I was also told about the tax-free element, which feels like you are putting "free money" into the pot! When I'm retired I want to be able to live life the way I live it now – eating out and going on holiday every now and again. But the biggest thing will hopefully be not worrying about money all the time; being able to afford the essentials but also the extra things that matter to me. I'm not sure yet about the actual percentage of my salary that will be – that will depend on so many things – whether I own a house and won't need to pay rent as I do at the moment, whether I'm married and have

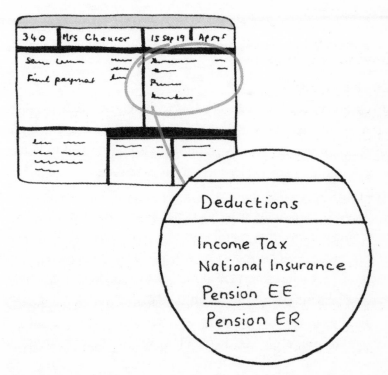

~ PAYSLIP ~

Deductions

Income Tax
National Insurance
Pension EE
Pension ER

children, where I live, what my health will be like and so on. Given all the unknowns it feels right to pay in as much as I can now to be as prepared as I can for whatever the future brings.'

Feel the benefit

As well as thinking about your pension, you or a family member or friend might be able to claim some benefits in later life. You may not realise this but:

- Thirty-six per cent of those entitled to Pension Credits don't claim the benefits that are due to them. That's £3.5 billion in unclaimed income that could help people who really need it.
- Nearly two out of five pensioners who are entitled to Pension Credit, on top of the state pension, do not claim it.

So, what are the benefits you might be entitled to, depending on your circumstances? Here are some of the key benefits you could apply for:

Pension credit
If you are an older person on a low income, you might be able to claim pension credit, which is a means-tested benefit. Depending on your household income, you might also be entitled to housing benefit and council tax reduction, or a rate rebate in Northern Ireland.

Women can claim pension credit once they've reached state pension age, even if they're still working. Your entitlement to housing benefit and council tax reduction will also be worked out differently once you've reached state pension age, so you might become entitled to these benefits even if you weren't before.

Because of the changes going on in the pension system, men can currently claim pension credit once they've reached the state pension age of a woman born on the same day as them – known as the pension credit qualifying age. Similarly to women, your entitlement to housing benefit and council tax reduction will also be worked out differently once you've reached this age, so you may be entitled to these benefits even if you weren't before.

If you get pension credit and you don't live in a care home, you'll be able to get help with fuel costs during very cold weather. Find out more about cold weather payments on Gov.uk.

Caring benefit

You might also be able to claim carer's allowance if you're acting as someone's carer and they're claiming certain benefits, such as personal independence payments or disability living allowance. If you're a carer for more than 35 hours a week, this can give you an extra £66.15 a week (2019/20 figures). If you receive carer's allowance, you automatically get national insurance credits as well. If you're not caring for someone every week full time, you might be able to get carer's credits, which fill in national insurance gaps and can ensure your entitlement to a state pension. This is if you're caring for more than 20 hours a week, but less than 35. Although carer's allowance isn't means tested, there is a cap on the amount you can earn from working and still be entitled to the benefit. In 2019/20, this meant you couldn't get carer's allowance if you earned over £123 a week after deductions. There's more about being a carer (millions of us are!) in Chapter Nine on friends and family later.

Travel concessions

In England, you're entitled to free bus travel when you are older. Many people absolutely prize their bus passes and reduced fare train deals – they expand your ability to travel the country/city as well as get around for practical purposes.

If you're a woman living in England, you can get free bus travel once you've reached your state pension age. If you're a man living in England, you can get free bus travel once you've reached the state pension age of a woman born on the same day as you. You might also get travel concessions on other sorts of public transport.

If you live in Wales or Scotland, you can get free bus travel if you're over 60 and may get cheaper rates on other sorts of public transport. For more information about travel concessions in Scotland, see the Transport Scotland website. In Northern Ireland, you can get free bus and train travel if you're over 60. For more information about travel concessions in Northern Ireland, see the NI Direct website.

A bus pass can take you the length and breadth of Britain for literally nothing. In 2013, Michael and Jacqui Burden took the 'world's cheapest holiday', arriving in Carlisle eight days after having left Exeter, having taken 28 buses to get there. More than 500 miles for free.

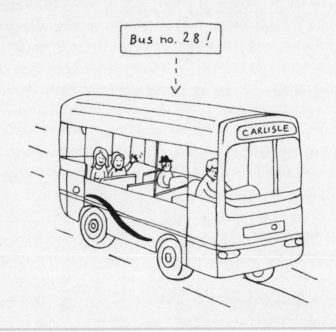

As well as this pass, at the time of writing there are still some benefits and concessions that older people can get – including a free TV licence if you're 75 or over (though I keep hearing about threatened withdrawal of this by the BBC); and potentially free NHS prescriptions and sight tests.

Paying for care

What is social care? We hear the term all the time in the news (usually accompanied by the word 'crisis'), but many people aren't sure exactly what it is, who provides it, and who pays for it.

In fact the term is a cover-all for a huge range of activity that helps care for people and protect them from harm, including vulnerable children as well as older adults. Social care also covers areas when you're older like help with washing, dressing, housework, making food and getting in and out of bed – and these can be provided in your home or in a care home, depending on your level of need.

Nearly 900,000 people over 65 received some form of social care in 2013/14. For about 400,000 people, this meant receiving care at home. Around 240,000 were in residential or nursing homes. Many of us tend to think – in an ageist way? – that most people who are much older are in care homes. But only 3 per cent of over-65s are receiving care in their own home, and only 2 per cent are in full-time care.

Local government has the main responsibility for providing care – from information and advice, through to assessment and monitoring people's needs and finances, and further to buying and monitoring the provision of care from a range of organisations.

People are sometimes surprised when they realise social care isn't free like NHS healthcare is. It's funded by people paying for their own care, by local government, and often a mix of the two.

To get publicly funded social care, your needs have to be high enough, and your means (i.e. how much you've got in savings, income and assets) low enough.

The social care system for older adults in England is particularly complicated and finding appropriate care for yourself or someone else can be something of a maze to navigate. There is a lot of variation depending on where you live, but getting care for yourself or someone else follows roughly the same process:

- You can refer yourself for a needs assessment, or make a referral for someone you know, as long as they agree to it. Your GP can also refer you.
- Your needs will be assessed to decide what care you need and to see what percentage, if any, you need to contribute to your care costs.
- There are slightly different thresholds above which you must pay for care around the country and these depend on the level of care you need.
- If you do need full-time residential care, the 'threshold' as of 2017 for paying for your own care in England and Northern Ireland was £23,250 (it's slightly higher in Scotland and Wales). That means if you have wealth, including savings and in this instance property, of more than this, you may have to pay your full costs. There are certain conditions in which you might be able to have your property excluded, such as if someone else is living at the property. If you own your home and are moving in to full-time care, you will probably have to pay your own care home costs.
- The value of your home is only taken in to account if you need to move to residential or nursing care. If you just need some help around the home, for example, it is excluded from your financial assessment.
- If the local authority decides to take payment from benefits, other payments or your bank accounts, they are still required by law to provide you with a certain amount each week, called a personal allowance. In 2017/18, this was £24.90 a week, to cover things like toiletries.
- If you decide to move to a more expensive care home than the one the council has suggested, the difference between what the council is

willing to pay and the cost of the home you choose must be covered. This is called a top-up, and is often paid by a third party, like a relative or partner.

- You don't have to sell your home to finance your care. But this may be the best option if you can't pay by any other means. Most councils will work with you to make sure you can meet costs in the way you choose. This might involve them covering care costs while you're selling your home or entering in to an agreement to recoup the money from the sale of your home after you die.

- You can't just give away your home or other savings/items of value to avoid paying for care. This is called deprivation of assets, and if you have given a gift or suddenly spent all your money on personal possessions solely to avoid care costs, the local authority may decide to include this as part of your financial assessment. Your local council will decide whether they think you have done this, mostly on the basis of whether you knew, or could have reasonably expected, to have to cover care costs shortly after you spent the money or gave the gift. If they think you have, they may include the value of these gifts or possessions bought to avoid care costs as part of your financial assessment.

Let's take the example of a real local authority. Shropshire Council follows this process:

- After you, or maybe a relative or GP, makes a referral for a needs assessment, the local authority determines what level of care it thinks you need, and what they can provide.

- To evaluate your needs, you'd need to attend a Shropshire Council 'Let's Talk Local' centre, where staff are trained to understand what your personal care needs are.

- If you decide you want to receive any care, you'd need to fill in a Financial Declaration form. This is the same whether you need a carer one day a week or are moving in to full-time care.

- The council then makes a decision on your contribution based on the wealth you hold, including property, unless there are special reasons why they shouldn't. This assessment would decide what you will pay, and what the council will, if any.

- You can choose to move in to the home that best suits your needs, but if it is more expensive than the one the Local Authority suggests, you will have to pay the difference. If the council says it will fund a room at one home in the centre of Shrewsbury, but instead you choose a room at a different home to be closer to family, you may have to pay more in top-up fees. Even if both residential homes are rated 'good' by the Care Quality Commission, your personal preference can mean significant cost.

If you have some care needs but can still just about get around yourself – make food, go to the loo and wash, for example – it's very unlikely any council will provide any free care unless you are in financial dire straits. This possibility, and the amount we'll have to potentially pay ourselves, feels daunting, and unless there's a very big and ongoing injection of cash into the social care system, doesn't look likely to change. This is one reason why being both as financially secure as possible and as healthy for as long as possible is important. The political climate may change, of course; the tax regime may change, and a cap may be put on the amount we have to contribute to our own costs of care. Worth thinking about when choosing who to vote for at the next election!

In 2017/18, there were more than 400,000 older people in residential homes and hundreds of thousands receiving care in their own home. Of the 400,000 people in residential homes, 176,000 (45 per cent) are self-funders who pay all their own costs and nearly 45,000 (11 per cent) pay some costs. Weekly costs in a care home average £617 (or £32,344 per year).

With the number of self-funders expected to increase, some parts of the finance industry are developing consumer products that can – as one financial provider put it – 'protect against the risk of catastrophic care costs on an individual level and can reduce the number of individuals falling back on state support on a society level'.

For example, Just (a financial services company) and Aviva (an insurance, savings and investment company) have developed a new product – an Immediate Needs Annuity (INA) – that they think could help. In exchange for an upfront premium, it provides a guaranteed income, for life, to pay just for care costs. They've developed it to help those who want to limit the risk of running out of money while they are in care or would like to ring-fence the amount of inheritance they can leave loved ones. The target market for this product is likely to be vulnerable customers – it's only offered on an advised basis through long-term care specialist independent financial advisors at the moment.

Whatever stage you find yourself at, in thinking about your own care needs or those of a relative, and how to pay for them, get advice on all the options beforehand. The Citizens Advice website is an absolute treasure trove of information on these areas and more. They also have advice centres where you can go and speak to a real person! Independent Age also have great factsheets on choosing a care home and paying for care among other areas on their website.

The press sometimes run awful stories about mismanagement and even abuse in care homes, but this is a rare occurrence and all care homes are regulated by the Care Quality Commission (CQC). It's their job to keep people safe from harm, abuse or neglect. As well as care homes they regulate hospitals, GPs, dentists, ambulances and mental health services, and care services that people receive in their own home. They publish all their findings online (cqc.org.uk), so when you choose care, you can see whether or not your choice of provider is rated 'outstanding', 'good', 'requires improvement' or 'inadequate'.

Thinking about the cost of care might be a long way down the road; if you keep fit and healthy and are lucky, you'll be able to manage without support for many years. And in those care-free years, as well as a pension, drawing down from other savings (or even continuing to build them up) is a great option for extra income.

Alternative ways to save

While I talk about various other savings options here, the key message is to really focus on your pension(s) as the savings vehicle to fund your later life and provide a regular source of income. It's more tax efficient and provides more of a guarantee of income.

But there are other ways to save and 'spread your bets' if you're in the lucky position to be able to put away more. To start with, pay off your debts before you start to save. Leaving your credit card debt to become mountainous and accumulate interest – plus putting money aside at the same time in an effort to save – doesn't make much sense.

Then, one of the simplest things you can do is put money away before it ever 'reaches you'. If you set up a direct debit to take out a certain amount every pay day, for example, you might not be tempted to skip a month or decrease the amount. You can save more than you think this way, and potentially without missing it. There are also new savings apps that 'round up' purchases and put the extra pennies and pounds into a savings or investment scheme – that could be another way to accumulate.

And where's the best place to put your carefully squirrelled-away funds? Well, the worst place to put any savings is under the mattress. As I'm sure is obvious to you, inflation shrinks the value of your money. That £100 you put under the mattress in 1990 is now worth about £50 in terms of today's buying power.

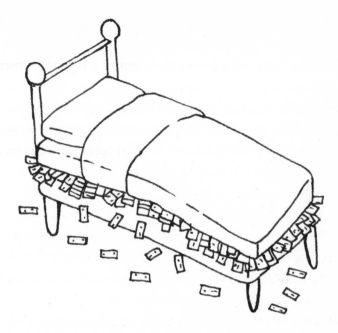

The place where most people save is of course in banks and building societies, where different deals on accounts can be found and there are plenty of value comparison websites to search for good deals on the best accounts. Having said that, at the time of writing, cash savings accounts have very low rates of interest – some in fact are at 0.0 per cent. You can't get lower than that without paying the bank for the pleasure of storing your money.

Where else to put the cash? Bonds could give you more income than a savings account but perhaps not as good a return as property. Next up are stocks and shares – over the long run, that is where your money might be best placed. While the value of cash erodes, and the housing bubble could burst, and while interest rates are low so a return from a straight savings account could be very small, equities have seen a fairly steady growth pattern, averaging at around 4.8 per cent a year between 1990 and 2015, notwithstanding the 2008 crash and smaller jitters on the world stock markets. So, a £100 deposit, with an average of 4.8 per cent interest over 25 years, would see you with £322.87 in your investment account.

Premium bonds, unlike savings accounts, don't accrue interest, but could be a fun way to save up to £50,000. Your bonds are entered into a monthly draw. ERNIE, the Electronic Random Number Indicator Equipment, is still in action, randomly picking winners from all existing bonds. You can win prizes from £25 to £1 million. The more bonds you buy, the higher the probability of winning prizes, and, if you've invested up to the maximum, you're likely to see some growth. Of course, there's no guarantee that you'll win anything, but your original investment is protected by the Treasury.

The main thing to think about with savings is to spread your bets – have a diverse range of pots if possible, balancing out your risk. Taking a bet and putting all your savings on cobalt and platinum increasing in value is very risky. You might take risks with investments if you are so inclined when you're younger, but as you get older, start reshaping your portfolio so you're more risk averse. Ultimately with saving for your great later life, the most sensible thing to do is to put more into your pension and ISA.

Should you use a financial advisor? Some people find this enormously helpful, getting qualified expert people to help with financial planning. But it can be a minefield. Some advisors are tied to a company or paid commission to recommend particular products. An independent financial advisor should only have the client's best interests at heart. They should be on the Financial Conduct Authority register of IFAs (you can check online). Understand up front what they will charge for their services and be clear about what you need from them. Pensions advice? Savings products? Mortgage advice? The Pensions Advisory Service website has clear guidance on how and when to choose an independent financial advisor.

Great expectations

If you've got children, and if you own a house or have some cash in the bank, they might be forgiven for thinking that when you pop your clogs, after the grief will come the inheritance. You will very likely be happy to pass on any wealth or assets you've accumulated to help them become more financially secure. And if your parents are alive you might wonder whether you will be left with some of *their* assets after they pass away. As we all live longer, people in their 20s and 30s now can expect to wait. If they receive an inheritance, it will be on average when they are 61! One investment company estimated that a third of people under 45 are relying on an inheritance to help them financially in later life, with some saying it will 'fund their retirement'. This may be the case for some, but similarly to the discussion above on levels of risk associated with different types of income, changes in house prices could easily impact on expectations, as could changes to inheritance tax (in 2019 this was at 40 per cent, after a tax-free threshold of £325,000), and whether or not people will need to sell their houses to pay for care. So, while some will benefit from a 'private transfer' of wealth from parents or other relatives, it's probably not the sole answer in terms of financial security for the majority of people – including many who are relying on it to fund their later life.

****

In summary, we have to seriously rethink our assumptions about being financially secure as we live for longer. The first step is to make some reasonable assumptions and calculate what financial resources you'll need to enjoy later life. It's very likely you haven't got enough saved yet, nor perhaps have plans on an ongoing basis to save. We all need to do this, and probably not think we can rely on the state pension as much as previous generations were able to. While many people do rely on it, the state pension acts more as a guard against absolute poverty than a source of funds to maintain the lifestyle you might expect. For most of us, that will mean simply working for longer (and that doesn't have to be a drag, as we'll discuss in the next chapter) and putting more into pensions and savings products. But there may be a range of other options as well – do you have or are you on the way to having housing assets? Might you be able to invest in stocks and shares? Have you considered other sources of income like starting your own business, or taking part in the 'gig economy' using an online platform to rent out a room in your house, for example?

A final, sure-fire alternative to having enough money in later life by working longer, investing and saving is buying a lottery ticket. The odds of winning the lottery are 1 in 45 million: at least 5,000 people have become millionaires through winning the lottery across the UK. But hey, if you play, you'll be helping good causes and you might even win a few bob back – if not a million!

5

NICE WORK IF YOU CAN GET IT

By now you've worked out that you've probably got more years of life left than you initially thought. But have you really considered what you're going to do with them? There are a range of factors to think about here, including what you really love doing, and how you'll fund it. A crucial decision to make is how long you want to work – what kind of work is right for you as you move through middle age to preparing for later life, and what learning and skills you'll need for it (yes – you heard that right – keeping on learning is going to be crucial).

If you're thinking about working for longer, you wouldn't be alone. Over-50s now make up nearly one-third (31 per cent) of the entire UK workforce, up from around one in five (21 per cent) in the early 1990s – and there were 10.3 million 'older workers' in October 2018. That's the equivalent of the entire population of Sweden.

Most people might say they 'work to live' rather than 'live to work'; in the last chapter I mentioned that working for longer (but perhaps in a different way) could really help both in terms of current living costs but also pension contributions and other ways of making sure you're financially secure. But money is not the only reason for working. If you've got a good-quality job, that can really add to your health and happiness as well as your wealth.

Would you agree with any of the statements on the next page?

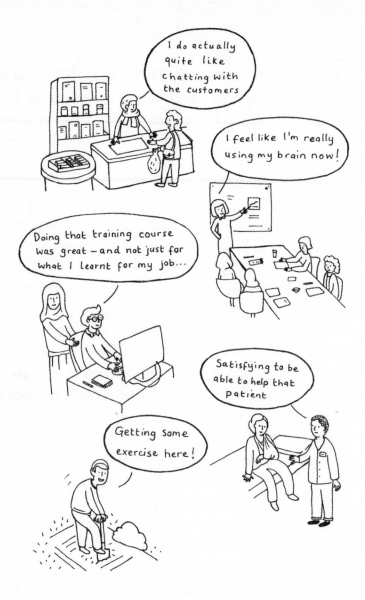

You might have your own thoughts about why work can be good. But being sociable and talking to colleagues, using your intelligence and learning new things, enjoying customer service or helping others, and even keeping physically active are all great reasons to stay working.

What is 'good work'? Well, the type of job that's 'good' for you is going to be different for everyone. And while money will be important, it isn't the only factor. In fact, we know that good work has similar ingredients for people of any age. It's about having flexibility, being supported by managers and getting on well with colleagues, about having choice and control over when, where and how you work. For most people, your work having value that's special to you is the thing that keeps you going. And for many, another key factor in good work is a sociable environment, with people of different ages working together, learning from each other, and not stereotyping by age.

But specifically, as you get older, some things do change. You're more likely to have a health condition or caring responsibility, and you'll need your employer to support you to manage your work and home life. Obvious things like time off for medical appointments, and small changes – like providing a headset if you work on the phone a lot – could be important, or even being able to use your mobile in work time if you're a carer and need to be in touch with your loved one.

Lots of people in middle age who are juggling home responsibilities as well tell us they can't wait to retire, but when you get under the skin of that statement, more often than not they mean they don't like their current job! And this is often because they feel trapped and have a sense that things can't change. It's a sad state of affairs to feel like that. But things can change. Training and development is as much for you as anyone else, as is getting a promotion. Lose that perception that 'if you haven't made it by 40 you're never going to make it', because this way of thinking needs to change radically.

In middle age or later life, these problems can feel worse. The stakes can seem higher if you 'make a fuss', and fears about losing pension entitlements or being made redundant, alongside the challenge of getting a new job, could be overwhelming.

What is a mid-life MOT?

You may be familiar with the concept of a health 'MOT' – the NHS health check that you can get every few years between the ages of 40 and 74. Recently, the government has been thinking about providing a more general MOT in middle age. This service would be aimed at those in their 40s and 50s and involve a discussion about your current situation and future options around health, finances, work and retirement, as well as your pension. Questions (some more existential than others) that could be posed at a 'mid-life MOT' might be:

- Do I want to retrain in a different industry?
- What do I want to do with my life, and how will I fund it?
- Do I want to, or need to, work again after I retire?
- Who in my family might need care in the near future, and what will I need to do to prepare for that?

As you're reading this book, you are clearly already on the journey of self-awareness when it comes to considering most or all of these questions and more; but face-to-face and personalised advice like this could be a boon. If mid-life MOTs become a reality and are offered on a widespread basis, take one up!

How working longer should work

If you're at least in part convinced that for a range of reasons working longer – or even going back to work once you've 'retired' – could be a really good choice, how can you make it happen? Changing your own mentality about working into later life is just one part of the picture. But how can you help make sure your employer supports you in doing this?

At the Centre for Ageing Better we've created the 'Age-Friendly Five' for employers: what they need to do to become age-friendly.

We tell them that having a diverse age range of staff is great for their business – older workers transfer vital knowledge and skills, and age diversity can better match the customer base they're serving. Mixed age workforces mean greater productivity because strengths and weaknesses are balanced – older workers draw on a lifetime of experience and younger workers can bring a fresh perspective. So what do they need to do, and how can you help them? Employers should:

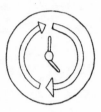

Be flexible about flexible working. This means they should offer more kinds of flexibility, manage it well and help people know their options. Know your rights about asking for flexibility if you need or want it, and work with your employer to find the best fit for you and the business.

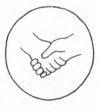

Hire age positively. I talk about this elsewhere – there is bias in recruiting older people and employers need to wipe this out! They should actively target candidates of all ages. If you think this is going on in your company or organisation, question it. And if you feel you have been discriminated because of your age, ask if age was a criterion in selection. Age discrimination is illegal and can be challenged.

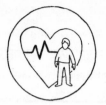

Ensure everyone has the health support they need. This means employers should have early and open conversations and make sure workers have access to support. Talk about your health with your employer at recruitment and your manager on an ongoing basis. If they are a good employer they should take an empathetic and supportive approach – helping you manage your health will mean you're more positive about working for them. You should never be penalised for disclosing a health condition.

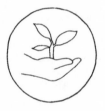

Encourage career development at all ages. No, you're not 'too old' to progress or skill up. Employers should make sure there are opportunities for people to develop their careers and plan for the future at mid-life and beyond. Be proactive about asking for and taking up development opportunities and challenge practices that seem to discount middle-aged or older employees when it comes to promotion and training.

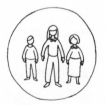

Create an age-positive culture. HR, talent managers, personnel, the people team; however they describe themselves, it's part of their job to try and create an 'age-positive' culture – to support interaction across ages, stop any signs of ageism, and make sure they are monitoring and measuring what's happening on age. How many flexible working requests have been made and how many granted? What's the age profile of applicants and successful candidates? What are they going to do to improve this if there's clearly a problem? Encourage your HR team to think about, and act on, creating an age-positive culture.

I focus on some of these areas more as the chapter goes on. This is a rallying cry for all of us in mid-life and beyond who might be classed as 'older workers' – we have the power to help change things for the better even if our employers haven't caught up yet. Help make the change and talk to your HR team and manager about the Age-Friendly Five!

The gig economy and self-employment

What is the 'gig economy'? Could gig jobs or self-employment offer the right kind of income and flexibility for you?

If you follow the news, you'd think that driving an Uber, letting out your room on Airbnb or running a pop-up falafel van is the main driver of the UK economy. The 'gig economy' sector is often defined as a sector in which people work on short-term, often zero-hour contracts, facilitated by technology such as phone apps, which allow you to expand your reach to a large consumer market. It's increasing but is still only 4.4 per cent of the workforce. It could be a good option for more income. Eleven per cent of Airbnb hosts are over 60 years old…

Self-employment, however, is a really growing phenomenon, particularly for people as they grow older. In 2017, 4.8 million people registered as self-employed, higher than at any point since records began. People are taking back control of their working lives by doing things like setting up their own business, working as a freelancer, or perhaps running a franchise.

But while this is a positive choice for many – you can be your own boss, after all – we know that some people actually become self-employed because of a lack of other options. If you can't get a good job in your area, setting yourself up as a handyman or hairdresser might seem like one of the few choices left to you. But the downsides of self-employment include no pension, sick or holiday pay or leave, insecurity, and perhaps a lack of contact with regular work colleagues. So, while being self-employed could be a great opportunity, think about:

- What it would mean for your income – particularly if your cash flow could be erratic – including your ability to put money aside for unexpected events (which perhaps becomes more and more important as you grow older).
- How you'll save into a pension, given you're not auto-enrolled into an occupational scheme by an employer.
- What would happen if you got sick or had an accident.
- Whether or not you have the skills and knowledge to do your own accounts and the other legal obligations of running a business, or have built in the costs to pay others to do this.

But having considered the risks, think about the benefits! There are potential massive upsides, and while you're not guaranteed success, there is some evidence that older entrepreneurs are more likely to have successful start-ups than younger people. There's also lots of support out there. UnLtd is an organisation that supports 'social entrepreneurs' – people who are working to improve the lives of others and make a positive impact in the places they live and work.

The support includes funding as well as advice. If you have a great idea, contact them!

Bad work

We've explored some of the benefits of staying in work for longer, and they also apply if you return to work after being unemployed or after 'retiring' from a different job. They're not just financial benefits but also to do with connecting with people, using your mind (and body), and clearly having something to get up for in the morning. But obviously not every job, all the time, is great. We live in the real world, not one full of stock photos of people sitting at desks or on construction sites perpetually sharing a joke and slapping each other on the back. And unless the work you do is good-quality work, it might not have the positive effects we're talking about – in fact, it could even be harmful.

So, what is 'bad work' and what can you do about it?

Lots of people are stuck in jobs where it feels like none of the quotes illustrated at the beginning of the chapter apply, nor are any of the 'Age-Friendly Five' followed. The work culture might be oppressive or very hierarchical – somewhere where staff aren't trusted, their ideas aren't listened to, and they don't have the power to make any decisions themselves. Bad jobs have no flexibility about the hours you work and are situations where your employer doesn't care about your health and indeed might frown on you taking time off for doctor's appointments. It could be about the job being insecure – older workers have seen the biggest decline in how secure they say they feel at work over the last 10 years. If you're working in a 'gig economy' type job or on a zero-hours contract, it might be that the positives on flexibility are outweighed by the negatives of having no sick or holiday pay. At their worst, bad jobs can be bad for your physical health as well as your state of mind.

Getting back into work

Lots of people find themselves out of work, and desperately want to get a job. In fact, there are an estimated 1 million people between 50 and the state pension age who would like to be in work but are not for a variety of reasons. One of the most common issues people talk about is the difficulty of combining being a carer for a spouse, parent or other loved one plus doing a full-time or even part-time work. Another is having a health problem or multiple health problems; worrying about potential employers being put off because of this and knowing that you'll need time off for medical appointments. Some health conditions make people worry that lots of travel to work or having to stand all day will aggravate their back pain or breathing problems. And some people who are depressed (perhaps in part because of being unwell) find the whole idea of applying for, then applying themselves to a job, an overwhelming prospect.

I'm painting a gloomy picture here – but you might know someone like this, and at times throughout our lives, any one of these reasons might apply to any one of us. I also find that when I've had periods of time out of work, gradually my confidence shrinks until I wonder if I have the skills needed to do jobs – even when, objectively, I know I'm qualified for them. I have to sit myself down and give myself a serious pep talk! So, here's some advice for people who find themselves in the tricky position of trying to get back into work while juggling other responsibilities, or health problems, or even think that applying online, for example, is just too complicated.

I am a full-time carer for my husband who is unwell, but I want to get back into work. What should I do?

Lots of people find themselves in this situation. They love their partner and are happy to look after them, but sometimes feel lonely and stuck. People may need the income but are certainly also looking for the friendship and mental stimulation that work can bring, as well as just a change of scene.

The key is to have the right conversations with potential employers. Talk about your need for flexibility from the outset. Many carers have health conditions themselves – and it's not impossible to manage caring responsibilities, health conditions and work, so don't write it off as an idea.

Recognise what value you can bring to workplaces. As a carer, what skills do you bring to a potential work environment? Patience, resilience to change, practical thinking, organisation skills? You have a legal right to ask for flexible working after you've been in a job for six months and many employers will take their responsibilities to offer flexibility to their employees seriously.

For some people, work isn't the right thing. While it might not boost your finances, the contribution you make to your family and community is equally valuable. And if you are caring for others, make sure you claim the benefits due to you. As mentioned in the 'funding it' chapter, many carers can claim a range of benefits and some people can claim National Insurance credits for looking after grandchildren. The Carers UK website is an invaluable source of information for carers and a place where you can connect with others in your situation.

The reason I lost my last job was because I was suffering with really bad back pain and that led to stress and depression. I felt my employer didn't support me and I just couldn't take it any more. I do want to be in work though!

This is such a common problem. In 2012, the Department of Health estimated that there were 15 million people with long-term conditions. In this case I'd say 'know your rights'. You have the right to request reasonable adjustments to manage a health condition from your employer. There's a government Access to Work scheme that exists as much for someone with diabetes as someone paralysed because they've been in a car crash.

It's also important not to hide things from a current or potential employer. Talk about any issues, such as your health, from an early stage. Give the employer the chance to act and know how to respond if they don't do what they should – including making reasonable adjustments like time off for medical appointments. It's not just about them, of course. Finding a way of getting in control and managing your health condition yourself is really important and there are charities as well as your local GP who can give you advice and support to do this.

I've applied for over 100 jobs and not got anywhere – it's getting me down.

You're not alone so don't take it personally! Seek help. There's support out there, and not just for younger people looking for work. The National Careers Service (look on Gov.uk) provides help with training and courses and has a 'skills health check' you can do. Bursaries and grants are often available for adult learners. Further Education colleges often offer subsidised training for people to reskill, and there are many community organisations that offer support on CV writing, interview training and presentation skills.

But whatever your personal skills and experience, we do know that there's ageism in recruitment of older workers. It's a scandal and deeply unfair that people will be ruled out by hiring managers just because of their age. In 2015 researchers at Anglia Ruskin University sent 1,800 companies two identical CVs, fundamentally different only in the dates of birth of the candidate. Surprise, surprise – employers invited the 'younger' applicant to an interview more than four times as often as the 'older' one.

We carried out our own survey to see if people felt they had been discriminated against by recruiters because of their age. It showed that, since turning 50, 14 per cent of over-50 employees believe they have been turned down for a job due to their age and nearly one in five (18 per cent) have or have considered hiding their age in job applications. Nearly half (46 per cent) think their age would disadvantage them in applying for a job and one in five think people see them as less capable due to their age.

We need to work to expose this blatantly ageist behaviour and put a stop to it. It shouldn't put any of us off in being confident in our hard-earned skills and abilities, and what, as older workers, we can offer to prospective employers.

Training and learning

Keeping up your skills and learning new ones are important to stay relevant in the workplace as well as just for your enjoyment – a commitment to professional development in whichever field you work in is essential.

As part of its commitment to get more older workers back into work, the Government recently set a target of 3 million more apprenticeships by 2020. While most people think of an apprenticeship as something solely for young people to learn a skill or trade, this is also a way for people later in life to retrain. Since 2015, Barclays has operated 'Bolder Apprenticeships', for example, aimed at widening participation in apprenticeships, including people who have been out of work for some time or spent most of their working life in other fields.

Even if you're not looking to change career trajectories, you should still be getting workplace training, whatever age you are. OECD data suggests that only Turkey does worse than the UK when it comes to learning in the workplace for older workers. People over 55 are significantly less likely to be offered training, even though they could be with the company for another 15 years or longer.

Out of the workplace, if you want to refresh your skills and learn something new, but haven't been to school, college or university in decades, there are still plenty of places you can go, and resources you can use. Here are some of them:

- The Workers' Educational Association provides thousands of courses around the country, and if you're in receipt of certain benefits, including Pension Guarantee Credit, these are subsidised. While you can take a class to brush up your maths or learn digital skills, you also might want to take 'Architectural Pottery' or '100 Years of Political Assassinations'! They're also looking for teachers and volunteers.
- Universities frequently offer evening or weekend classes, with people from all ages participating. These can range from language classes to music and drama lessons. You don't necessarily have to physically attend classes either. Online courses are becoming a great way for people to commit to learning and can often be more flexible than other types of education. FutureLearn and OpenLearn, both owned by the Open University, are good places to start. They provide thousands of hours of free learning online, with a large range of possible areas to focus on including business- and career-related courses.

- Local libraries frequently offer classes aimed at people who want to improve their digital skills. They might also offer classes or have discussion groups about other areas such as family genealogy or local history.
- If you're retired, there's no reason why you can't attend university full-time if you want to (and can afford to). If you want to re-engage with the joyful challenge of intellectual stimulation, give structure to your days and weeks, learn new skills and make new friends, maybe getting that degree you always wanted is still possible.
- If you're interested in learning for the fun of it when retired rather than working towards a formal qualification, check out the University of the Third Age (U3A). There are 1000 local 'universities' around the country with a total of 400,000 members who share skills and knowledge. Members often have teaching experience themselves. Membership is usually around £35 or less and you could find yourself learning (or teaching) music, crafts, cooking, history and a host of other subjects and skills with others.

Retirement

In our inbox at the Centre for Ageing Better, every now and again we get the simple question:

When should I retire?
You know that in almost all jobs there's no set retirement age. You should not be in receipt of a gold-plated carriage clock and a wave goodbye from the boss the moment you turn 65. And you know that whether it's part-time or full-time, every year you spend working after the age of 65 has serious financial benefits as well as many others. Even if you're in a job where there is a set retirement age, there's nothing stopping you carrying on working in a different job or setting yourself up as self-employed.

But if you are set on stopping working altogether, the simple answer to the 'when should I retire' question is: it's up to you.

Of course, making that decision an informed one is the best way to go about it. A vague idea of retirement being a land of milk and honey in the distance and picking a date at random is probably not the best approach...

Here are the key things to think about to inform that decision:

- Will I have enough money to cover living expenses, travel and hobbies, any spending on rent or my home, and possible costs of care? Do I know how my financial outgoings will change over time? What is my annual income and expenditure likely to be, taking into account state and other pensions?

- Have I got the friends, family and social links I will need to keep me connected – or am I mainly relying on work for people to talk to and hang out with?

- How might retirement change my relationship with my partner? If they work, when are they planning to retire? Should we both talk about how we're going to feel about potentially spending lots more time together?

- Have I thought about what I will do with my life – do I have hobbies I want to pursue more, or are there volunteering opportunities I could take up? Is there something I've always wanted to learn about but haven't had the time?

Here at the Centre for Ageing Better we have been working with the Calouste Gulbenkian Foundation to support a group called the 'Transitions in Later Life' (TILL) projects. The folk running these projects meet regularly to share their knowledge about how to help people through big life changes like retirement. TILL members come from many different types of organisations – including a health trust, charities, and organisations that focus on psychology and counselling – but what they all have in common is experience in using therapeutic approaches to help individuals manage what can sometimes be very challenging changes. Many of them employ practitioners and trainers in psychotherapy disciplines like CBT (Cognitive Behavioural Therapy) and mindfulness.

In their work with people going through retirement, they say there's often a sudden vacuum – a feeling of being destabilised, followed by what they call 'The Grab'. Reaching for anything to fill the vacuum left by not working: waxing the kitchen table three times in a year; volunteering for anything and everything; deciding to become an accomplished watercolourist despite never having picked up a paintbrush in your life. The Grab, says the TILL gang, is not a true response to the vacuum, it's a sign that your work was so overwhelming that you didn't manage to get to the holy grail of 'work-life balance' and find out what gives you joy before you retire. Their advice is in five parts:

1. Long before you retire, nurture your creativity and interests. Over 40 per cent of full-time workers (about 9 million people) also volunteer at least once a year, and millions of us have hobbies and interests we love. If work is your life, consider how to mix it up more before you stop the nine to five.

2. Think about whether or not you really need to retire abruptly, from permanent full-time work to no work at all. You could work for fewer hours or think about taking a break to do something you want like study or travel before returning to work.

3. Have a conversation with people who have gone through retirement, so you hear first-hand about both the great opportunities and the pitfalls, and how others have dealt with them.

4. Be conscious and think about what you do and don't want and talk to others about it – have the conversation and set expectations early on.

You might not want to look after your grandchildren five days a week, for example, but there could be unspoken expectations from your grown-up children that you will help out more.

5. Sit out periods of difficulty or seek help – there is no compulsion to fill your life with activity and force yourself to be positive if you don't feel that way. Accepting that retirement can sometimes be a hard transition can be an important step in adjusting to the change.

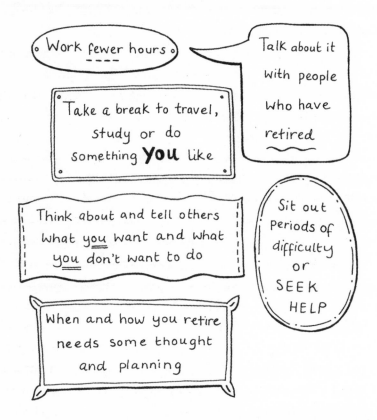

Since 2011, it's been illegal for most companies to force their employees to retire at a certain age. But there are exceptions. In some physically or mentally demanding jobs, like working as a firefighter, people have to retire at 60. The police and the armed forces are also exempt – they too have a compulsory retirement age set at 60. The law on no default retirement age also doesn't apply if there's an unclear relationship between the employer and employee. For example, law partners can be made to retire from their firm because they are not technically employees. And some other institutions have successfully made a case to keep a retirement age, which many might think unfair. Both Oxford and Cambridge universities, for example, enforce a retirement age so they can 'keep their global reputation and diversify their workforces'. Academics at Oxford have to retire by 68 and those at Cambridge currently have to hang up their gowns at 67.

Whether you're a builder, a baker or an interior designer, when and how to retire needs some thought and planning. Some enlightened employers provide help in the form of retirement courses. Here's Nora's story:

'My name is Nora Doleman, I've been nursing for over 50 years. I was asked if I'd like to go to a training programme around transition from working to either stepping down to part-time or continue to work into older years. I didn't know what to expect but it was a very positive thing that happened in my life. It opened up a whole bunch of conversations between people we didn't know and actually that helped every single one of us to sit our husbands down and just say, "What are we going to do? What do you think? What plans have you got?" We never really talked about the "What ifs" and what should we do or where we'll live, will we move? Will we stay where we are?

'I suppose I will retire someday but I never really thought about it until I went on that course and I think I've changed since then. It used to worry me, I used to think "What am I going to do when I can't do my job any more?" but I think it broke down a lot of emotional barriers, that are either perceived or real because we all think we haven't got any hang-ups about things but we do, we just don't give it a name, we don't talk about it, therefore it doesn't exist, so it gives you that strength to think about what you're going to do and actually talk about it.'

Sudden retirement – looking over the cliff edge

Our recent research showed that one in five people who retired in the last five years found it difficult, and only around half (56 per cent) of the people planning to retire in the next five years were looking forward to it. People were worried about managing their money (41 per cent), feeling bored (33 per cent) and missing their social connections from work (32 per cent). Nearly a quarter worried about losing their purpose (24 per cent). One in four people who have retired return to some form of paid work. More than a third wanted more advice about transitioning from work to retirement.

So, there's a lot to think about in terms of working longer, if and when you want to retire, and what that transition into retirement might look like. To summarise some of the key points:

- Most of us will need to carry on working for longer, to make sure that we have financial security for our long and great later lives, but we shouldn't see this as a drag. Work, if it's good work, can be fulfilling intellectually and/or physically, can give us friends and everyday social connection, give us a sense of pride and achievement, and make us feel like we're contributing to society, and to the economy.

- But bad work, or being out of work, can actually be harmful, and there's help out there to get into work and to choose the job that's right for you. This includes work with the flexibility you need to live in the way you want – for example, if you're caring for others or want to work fewer hours in a less stressful environment. It's up to you as well to learn and keep up your skills, present your experience and talents in a compelling way, and be resilient when there are knockbacks.

- Break the idea that at 65 (or younger) you will down tools for ever. Many who retire miss work and want to get back into it, and many who dream of retirement fervently do so because they just don't like their current job. You don't ever need to 'retire'!

- But if and when you do stop work for good, think about what that transition is going to look like and prepare well in advance. Think about the impact on your finances, relationships, and what you'll do to fill your time.

Volunteering

When you don't want to carry on working, what can give you meaning and purpose? Many people have the ageist assumption that most, if not all, of the people who volunteer in Britain are 'old ladies'. In fact, people of all ages volunteer and many of you will already be doing this. You might already know the pleasure and fulfilment it brings to help others or do unpaid work for a cause you believe in. About 40 per cent of people across the country do some kind of formal volunteering, and even more (53 per cent) report that they try to be good neighbours, doing small acts of kindness on a regular basis. But indeed, our extra years of life give us the potential to spend more time giving back and contributing to our community – and two-thirds of people who have retired make volunteering a part of their life.

I spoke with Shaun Delaney from the National Council for Volunteering Organisations and asked him what advice he would give to someone considering being a volunteer:

'The first thing to consider – and many people don't – is that volunteering's definitely a two-way thing. People's motivation to volunteer is wonderful – to help other people or the environment, or work for a cause they believe in. But if you consider what you want to get from it personally and then choose the volunteering activity that will fulfil your needs, it's much more likely to be a positive experience. Do you want to get new skills, for example, meet new people, create structure for your days or even see different parts of the world? I realise that this is a different way of thinking – to think about what you want. Beneficiaries are a huge part of the purpose of volunteering but give yourself permission to think about what you want to get out of it too. And there are thousands of possible roles, and this can be overwhelming, so being clear about what you want to get out of it will help you choose.

'Then – what excites you? Volunteering is really personal. Does the idea of cleaning out the local canal turn you on? Would fundraising for the hospice that gave such love and care for your grandad in his last years help you feel like you're giving back? Are you passionate about helping young people gain new skills? That will of course help narrow down the search even further. And of course, the flip side of that is what you're not so great at. Don't volunteer with the girl guides if you don't like being with kids so much!

'If you're kicking off volunteering for the first time, we know that when people develop habits early on they stick through life. So, starting early could be better – if you leave it until retirement it actually could be quite daunting. So, my best advice is, if you start volunteering before you retire, you'll have a better understanding of what it involves.

'How do you find the volunteering opportunities? There are many ways.

- If you're comfortable searching online, go through the NCVO website and the National DO IT website (see Top Resources).
- A local organisation might spring to mind – like a local hospice or scout group. Pick up the phone and give them a call to ask about volunteering roles.
- Chat to friends and family. It's very British not to talk about it, but most people have secret volunteers in their friends and family circle. They could put you in touch with the organisations they volunteer for.

- If you've got links to a faith organisation, they will often be grateful for volunteers from the congregation.
- Lots of counties and boroughs have some sort of volunteer centre and they often have drop-in sessions – details can be found at the library, tourist information and council website.

'Then if it's your first time, go easy. Go along for a day or session to see what it's like – start gradually without too big a commitment to yourself or the organisation.

'But you don't have to call yourself a volunteer if that sounds off-putting or formal. Some people would just call it "helping out" or a hobby – supporting their grandkids' scout group – getting involved – whatever. The definition is up to you.'

There are some people who think that volunteering is not for them – in fact, people who are less well-off, have fewer social connections and are less active in their lives would benefit most from contributing to their community, but they are the group that (formally) volunteers the least. There has been lots of government and voluntary sector attention on encouraging young people to volunteer; the time is right for a greater focus on helping all people in later life contribute to their communities. So, get out there and take part!

Digital

Should we all be online? Do you know the right way up to hold an iPad? (Digital savants will know that was a trick question.) Do you feel you've missed the digital revolution and don't know where to start?

The chart overleaf shows what percentage of every age group is not online. As you might expect, younger people are much more likely to be online than older groups, but there's also a big divide by gender. If you're over 75, you are much less likely to be online if you are a woman.

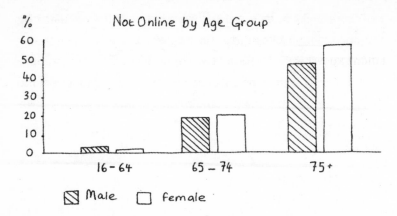

In a recent Centre for Ageing Better/Good Things Foundation report, we listened to experiences of people who just didn't go online, and people gave a range of reasons for never using the internet. Some said that as they hadn't been working outside of their home, they had never needed to use the internet. By the time it was introduced to them by children or grandchildren, they felt too stuck in their ways to learn something so different. Fear and misunderstanding of computers also meant that some didn't want to go online. One lady commented that 'The computer to me was just something that I dusted'.

But of course for you, or more likely your older relatives or friends, there's still time to learn. Some older people have spoken about the benefits of getting online – helping keep in touch with people and feeling less lonely. One person we interviewed, Bob (86), started using the internet with the help of his local online centre. Many online centres are based in your town centre library (or if not there, the library staff should be able to tell you where to find it). If you're looking for someone else, all the details for online centres are online.

'Every time I looked at the television, if I wanted to buy something or find something, I had to be online. I asked myself, "How do I get in touch with Amazon if I don't have a computer?"

'Being online has opened up a whole new world for me. I like being able to do things like banking, paying gas bills, and learning things I didn't know before – especially watching videos about engineering.

'What really helped me get online was having someone take me through things slowly, one-to-one, giving me time to go at my own pace and ask questions. I tried computer classes at night school, but they moved too quickly.'

Many of you will be familiar with some or all of the ways you can use the internet. If you have friends or family who need persuading, a list of everything they could do online might be a bit overwhelming and might actually put people off. It's better if you start with what the person actually wants to do then find the way digital can enable that – like Bob thinking about shopping online. But once people do start using the internet, there really is a world of opportunity and it's growing all the time – including:

- Keeping in touch – as well as face-to-face meeting and talking on the phone, services like Skype and FaceTime allow you to see and speak to friends and relatives wherever they are – and they are free.

- Getting healthcare – this is an area that's evolving rapidly. GP at Hand is a service offered in some areas that allows you to have a doctor's appointment via video on your smartphone. You have to change your registered NHS GP practice to GP at Hand to enable this. Most GP surgeries also now have online bookings for appointments, ways you can request repeat prescriptions digitally, and you should also be able to see your medical record online. There are also repeat prescription services that deliver to your door like Pharmacy2U. As well as this, there are thousands of health apps that can help you, ranging from blood glucose trackers for people with diabetes to exercise apps that ping you reminders to get up and stretch your legs if you've been sitting down for too long.

- Shopping and getting the best deals. The average person could save up to £744 per year by being online – so perhaps a good reason to use the internet and not miss out on good deals! This includes shopping for holidays as well as groceries, clothes, and almost anything else. You might think the demise of the high street is a shame – and I too prefer to buy food and clothes I can see in real life rather than on a screen – but the price and convenience of virtual buying are great positives.

- Paying bills and receiving benefits – whether you want to pay bills online or not, many companies and local authorities now push you into doing this 'by default'. If you're not comfortable doing this online, insist that you should be able to pay in the way that suits you. Get help from online centres locally if you are unsure about how to go about this.

- Searching for and applying for jobs. Remember the days of pages and pages of classified ads in nine-point type at the back of the papers? As well as the buy-and-sell and lonely hearts, that's where the job ads were. Again, jobs are almost exclusively advertised online now, so if you're looking for work, finding ways to search the recruitment sites and newspaper job pages as well as completing applications online (and sending letters of application/CVs via email) has become an essential skill.

- Finding out about local services and what's going on in your community. From bin collection to blue badges, to concerts, community groups, free film screenings, yoga classes, bake sales (I could go on) – the internet's got information on them all. As well as your local council website, local Facebook groups are often a huge store of information (and opinion, and advice) about what you can do and get involved with locally.

If you have a disability, it's possible to make adjustments so that you can enjoy the same access to the internet as everyone else:

- You can use voice recognition software like Dragon (or just use the voice feature on your phone, tablet or PC if it has one). There are programmes that type the words you say out loud, so you don't have to fiddle around with a keyboard, which is especially helpful for people with arthritis.
- If you have trouble seeing the screen, you can adjust the text size easily, so you can read it without glasses.
- Laptop tracking pads are notoriously tricky, and if you find them too difficult, you can always buy a separate mouse for your laptop – many people prefer this whether disabled or not.
- Ability Net has some excellent resources to help people use the internet more easily, including how to adjust the settings on your computer.

But do you want all this?

You might actually want to chat to a real, physical pharmacist who's right in front of you. You choose if the digital world is right for you. If it's not right for you or a parent/grandparent now, it might be in the future. Right now, you might see your daughter face-to-face, but what if in the future she moves and you want to keep in frequent contact? Ask yourself: are you able, or prepared, to respond to changes around you? Being digitally able could give you a safety net. And you don't have to learn everything at once. No need to feel like a failure if you haven't grasped Instagram instantly or don't know what the heck WhatsApp is! (In case you don't know, Instagram is for photo sharing and WhatsApp for having one-to-one chats in real time – known as instant messaging – and for group conversations. They're both available online or as apps.)

These places can help you, your friends and family become more digitally aware:

- UK online centres
- Local Age UKs

- Local libraries
- Housing Association if you're a social resident

Many young and adult children set out to help parents and grandparents get online and use the internet in a way that's going to make life easier, perhaps using some of the features I outlined above. The key things to remember if you're trying to help someone older are: be patient, don't rush, keep repeating how to do things, and don't be tempted to take the device off them and do it yourself! Don't be hard on yourself if you're struggling to help them or they need more help than you can give – it's not always easy. As I've noted above, there are online centres and other help you can tell them about.

Spot the scammers

Online scams are something that can affect people at any age, and the scammers are becoming very sophisticated. Some fraudulent emails look very realistic. Follow the advice underneath on how to tell real emails from the fake online:

- You don't remember ordering a vintage deer horn chandelier, so you click on the link you have been sent to query the purchase...
- Read carefully what your bank says about how it will contact you and obviously don't respond to any contact that isn't their normal protocol.
- Email items that seem to promise a refund or tell you you've overpaid or are owed tax are often fake.
- Find information from Citizens Advice or Age UK if you're unsure. They have expert knowledge and advice on how to spot a scam – and that includes phone fraudsters as well as dodgy door-to-door scammers.

This chapter has covered a lot of aspects, all with the central theme of how you're going to fill your time in the great extra years you've got ahead. From working through to retiring, learning more, volunteering, and using the internet to do a range of tasks and fun things, I still of course haven't covered (and couldn't cover) the vast choice of what you could spend your time doing. If you have fully or partly stopped working, the dream and reality of what you want to do will be entirely individual to you. The important thing to do is plan ahead. Be realistic about what it might take. If you want to spend years on a yacht, you'll need the wherewithal. Gardening for Britain might mean you need to be in good shape (and gardening can of course help with that). Your dream, for example, of volunteering and giving back to the community could be best started before you retire. Of course, you could just kick back and watch the telly. According to the ONS, enjoying mass media is by far our favourite thing to do in our spare time – on average we spend 16 hours a week watching TV, reading or listening to the radio. Hobbies like stamp collecting (still a favourite for many!), painting and writing poetry take up four hours a week.

What's your wish list? Mine probably includes a mix of part-time work, volunteering, gardening, travel, cooking and writing. Really interesting possible courses like foraging and wild food walks also catch my eye.

Whatever you decide, take the opportunity to make your later years as fulfilling as possible. But as well as the financial means to 'live the dream', you need to be in the best possible health you can be, and the next chapter explores how to stay well, and manage any health conditions you might have or get as you get older.

6

FIT AS A FIDDLE OR GOOD ENOUGH HEALTH?

To have an amazing longer life, there's one major factor that people rate above all others: health. We want to be able to get out and travel, work, enjoy our hobbies, see our friends and family, and obviously be able to do very basic things like get out of bed, go to the loo, and eat. We hope to be healthy right to the end.

But perhaps fatalistically, we expect to have one or more diseases, illnesses, long-term conditions – call them what you will. We expect that we will get arthritis, that our vision and hearing will fail, that we may get heart disease, cancer or dementia. In fact, if you're reading this and you're in your 50s and 60s or beyond, you may already have at least one condition. And it's true that the prevalence of long-term conditions like heart disease and arthritis is higher in people over 50. On average men will live 16 of their final years of life with multiple conditions, and women 20. Living in pain and discomfort at any time is miserable, but having years of it when you're older is not the best way to end a life well lived.

The myths

What makes us ill as we age? Is illness inevitable? Let's blow the dust off some of the myths and preconceptions and look at the facts:

Everyone gets ill when they're older – and if you're very old, it's inevitable you'll be very ill and frail.

This just isn't true. While 58 per cent of people over 50 have one long-term condition, and 43 per cent of people have two or more, not all older people are frail. Sixty per cent of 70-year-olds and 20 per cent of people who are 90 are 'fit', according to the National Clinical Director for older people. This means that they are robust, and either healthy or successfully managing health conditions. They are able to do most everyday activities independently.

Type 2 diabetes runs in families, so if you've got a family history of it you'll definitely get it sooner or later – there's nothing you can do about it.

Another myth to be busted. Your chances of getting Type 2 diabetes do increase by 15 per cent if one of your parents has it, and if you're from a South Asian background your risk is much higher, but you can still prevent it or at least delay when it starts by keeping your weight down and doing exercise.

Millions of people have dementia, and it's not preventable.

People are really worried about dementia. It's understandable – losing our memories, not recognising people we love, and losing our sense of self is a frightening thought. In fact, we're worried about it more than other diseases or health problems we're on average more likely to get. You might think that millions of people are living with dementia in the UK. But the actual number of people with the condition is around 850,000. And the British Social Attitudes survey shows that over a quarter of people (27 per cent) don't think there is anything you can do to reduce your risk of getting dementia. Sometimes there is. A recent long-term study has found that exercise and eating healthily are among the factors that might reduce your chance of getting dementia. There's more on this subject later in the chapter.

Once you lose your strength you'll never get it back.
It's true that muscles start to waste as you get older – every decade from 40 onwards you lose around 8 per cent of your muscle mass. But the great news is that this loss of power is reversible – doing strength and balance exercises like playing badminton or golf, practising tai chi or using weights and other machines at the gym will build muscle mass and bone strength, and help with balance. It's as important as aerobic exercise for your long-term health.

Types of illness

In my 'Top 10' at the beginning, I talked about three specific things that would make a huge difference: stopping smoking, not being overweight, and being more physically active, including doing a couple of sessions of strength and balance training a week ('standing on one leg'!). Each of these is vitally important in preventing ill health, delaying the onset of disease, and managing your health if you become ill.

Here's a run-through of the most common health conditions we experience as we get older: what causes them, how to prevent or delay getting them, including the vital points about weight and exercise above, and the importance of managing the condition well if you have it. In the section about dementia, given our particular fear of getting it, there's more on how to stave it off and some key facts to remember about the condition, from the Dementia Friends movement.

Type 2 diabetes

Type 2 diabetes is a condition where your body stops being able to regulate its own insulin levels – and insulin is the key to allowing your cells to gain energy from the food we eat. There are around 4 million people living with the condition across the UK, up from 1.8 million 20 years ago. As your body can't get enough glucose into your cells, a common symptom of Type 2 diabetes is feeling very tired. Other symptoms include needing to urinate a lot, feeling extremely thirsty, cuts and grazes healing slowly, and getting infections like thrush.

A lot of people don't get any symptoms, or they don't notice them. Some people don't think the symptoms are important, so don't ask for help. This means that some people live with Type 2 diabetes for up to 10 years before being diagnosed.

Over a long period of time, high glucose levels in your blood can seriously damage your heart, your eyes, your feet and your kidneys. But, with the right treatment and care, the effects of diabetes and high glucose levels can be managed. So, if you've got any of these symptoms, see a doctor as soon as possible.

There are different ways of treating Type 2 diabetes. Some people can manage it by healthier eating, being more active and losing weight. Eventually most people will need medication to bring their blood glucose down to a safe level – but you can delay this point for many years if you have great control over your diet and activity levels. It's worth saying, by the way, that there are a lot of misconceptions about Type 2 diabetes out there, and around a tenth of cases are seen in apparently slim and healthy people.

In a groundbreaking trial funded by Diabetes UK, Professor Roy Taylor of Newcastle University put people who had been recently diagnosed with Type 2 diabetes on a strict 800-calorie-a-day diet. Almost half of the participants, and particularly those who lost a lot of weight, put their diabetes into remission – effectively reversing it. This could have major implications for anyone newly diagnosed, but it's still the case that for the majority of people, diabetes is a lifelong and progressive condition.

Given how serious Type 2 diabetes can be in its later stages – it's the leading cause of amputation in Britain, for example, mainly because of foot ulcers that haven't healed – prevention, and self-management, are critical. Of course, the key to preventing its development lies in eating a healthy diet and doing plenty of exercise: being overweight or obese is the biggest risk factor in developing Type 2 diabetes. Reducing your body weight by just 5 per cent and staying active can halve your chances of getting the condition. Carrying extra weight around your stomach can be particularly harmful – so watch your waistline.

There's lots of debate around low-carb diets at the moment. While some people swear by them for weight loss and Type 2 diabetes control, the official advice is still to have a healthy balanced diet and not to go to extremes of low (or high) levels of carbohydrates.

Although diet and exercise are useful in preventing Type 2 diabetes, they can also help people who already have the condition to control their symptoms. Diabetes UK and the NHS website provide lots of information and DUK has support groups, a helpline and a host of other resources to help people understand and reduce their risk of getting it, and supporting people living with all types of diabetes.

Pat Scully, aged 58 and living in Cornwall, is on a mission to prove you can prevent Type 2 diabetes. Pat went from having a diagnosis of pre-diabetes to having lower blood glucose levels, well within the normal range. He beat diabetes by attending a Cornwall Healthy Weight course, lost four stone in a year, and is determined to keep healthy, and is even doing a long awareness-raising cycle ride for charity Diabetes UK. Pat's willpower is inspiring:

'I love my grub – I'm the kind of person who will have two steaks instead of one. I knew I was overweight, but I didn't know how to go about tackling it until I went on the course. Education is so important. Now I am down to 10 stone 4 pounds, I weigh myself every day, keep a food diary, and have an app to check what I'm eating. I also cycle, go to the gym, and go for long walks with my partner, Anne. I want people to know that it's possible to make lasting changes and avoid a diagnosis of Type 2 diabetes.'

Heart disease

Heart conditions and problems come in many forms, broadly called cardiovascular disease. This covers blocked arteries, angina and problems with the blood vessels of the heart. In the UK, men are more likely than women to suffer from heart conditions, and older people are more likely to develop heart disease than younger people. There are an estimated 7 million people in the UK with some form of heart disease.

Some people have a family history of heart disease, but as with other conditions, many cardiovascular diseases are preventable with lifestyle changes. I think you can guess the next bit: stopping smoking and reducing drinking can help reduce your risk, as can eating healthy food and exercising regularly. Those at the highest risk of heart disease are people with other health conditions such as diabetes, high blood pressure or high cholesterol, and they should be particularly conscious of their heart health.

For heart disease, Type 2 diabetes and other elements of your health, remember to take advantage of the free NHS health check offered to 40- to 74-year-olds in England, and 40- to 64-year-olds in Scotland. Although Wales does not currently offer these checks proactively, you can ask for one. Catching heart disease early can prevent heart attacks, strokes and serious disability, so paying attention now has the potential to reduce your chance of more serious illness in the years to come.

The British Heart Foundation has extensive information on how to cope if you've been affected by heart disease and lists the steps you can take to prevent heart problems. As with any of these health problems, also talk to your GP about prevention and management.

Super statins

After considerable nagging from my GP, I started taking statins a couple of years ago. From a perilous cholesterol level of over eight, my levels have reduced to under five! Different types of statins are used to treat the same thing: high levels of 'bad' cholesterol. If your cholesterol levels are too high, fatty deposits can block your arteries and cause heart disease, stroke or heart attacks. Statins to treat this are the most commonly prescribed medications in the UK, with about 7 million people taking them each day. Some people report side effects such as aching muscles and leg pain; you might need to change the statin until you find one that suits you, in discussion with your GP (this happened to me for a few months when I started taking them). Once you've been prescribed a statin, you'll usually have to take one a day for the rest of your life, but it's worth it – evidence has proven that long-term statin use can prevent life-threatening conditions.

Cancer

Cancer Research UK estimates that nearly 40 per cent of cancers are preventable, and there are plenty of steps you can take now to reduce your risk of developing most kinds of cancer. At the risk of sounding like a broken record, lifestyle factors, such as losing weight and keeping fit, are important, as is not smoking and reducing the amount of alcohol you drink.

Top tips on stopping smoking

If you or someone you know still smokes, despite the widespread knowledge of its harm and the gruesome photos of diseased organs on packs, here are some tips for quitting:

- You can try going cold turkey. This works for some people, but not others. You still need the determination and a positive attitude to stop, and to not be put off by times when you've tried and failed.

- If you're reaching for nicotine replacement like chewing gum, I'm afraid that this hasn't got any higher rate of success than 'cold turkey' if you try it on its own without professional support. One large study suggested this was because people don't know how much to take/use. However, if you do use it with advice from your GP or pharmacist (who might suggest, for example, combining a slow-release patch with a fast-release product like gum or nasal spray), this might increase your chance of quitting.

- E-cigarettes are becoming a very popular alternative to smoking tobacco, and lots of people are using them as an aid to quitting. Public Health England's evidence review found that vaping and e-cigarettes are much safer than cigarette smoking. Nevertheless, they're a relatively new product, so we won't know if there are long-term effects for some time, and more research is needed. Vaping can be really useful in helping smokers find an alternative that's far less risky than cigarettes. As with other nicotine replacements, you increase your chances of success if you get some advice and support.

- The best approach by far is to get a combination of support and medication. This could include counselling or 'stop smoking' groups with trained advisors, prescription medication to reduce cravings, and prompts that keep your motivation high such as an email and text support programme. If you have a local 'stop smoking' service, contact them now.

Bowel, breast and cervical cancer screenings are available through the NHS and can find cancers before symptoms develop, and in some cases prevent cancers from developing in the first place. Finding cancer at an early stage means treatment is more likely to be successful. Though anyone can be affected by it, the risk of cancer increases as we get older. You can find more information on what's available to you and at what age on the NHS website. Screening saves lives from cancer, but also has harms, so read the information you get with your invitation carefully to help you decide whether or not to take part in cancer screening.

If several close family members have had cancer, you may be more likely to get the disease. But most cancers aren't due to inherited risk. If you're worried that you might be at increased risk, speak to your doctor, who will be able to help.

If you are diagnosed with cancer, there are plenty of type-specific support groups around, but for general support and information on cancer generally, Cancer Research UK has great resources on preventing, treating and managing your life with cancer. Macmillan Cancer Support can provide practical support, including specialist nurses who are trained to answer your questions.

Many people think a diagnosis of cancer is a death sentence, but this isn't necessarily true. Cancer survival has doubled since the 1970s. Some people are redefining cancers as a long-term condition; with breast or prostate cancer, for example, around 80 per cent of people can expect to survive for at least 10 years after diagnosis and treatment.

Stroke

A stroke – sometimes known as a 'brain attack' – is when the blood supply to part of your brain is cut off. A stroke can happen to anyone, but you're more likely to have one the older you get. They often happen to people with existing health conditions like diabetes, high blood pressure or high cholesterol. Recovery from a stroke can be difficult, so avoiding a stroke or acting quickly means that you could avoid a long recovery period.

Acting FAST

Acting quickly can help reduce the impact the stroke will have on somebody, so it's important to know the signs that someone has had a stroke and needs assistance. The Stroke Association created and has done lots to publicise the acronym FAST:

- Face: is the person's face drooping on one side, or are they having trouble controlling their facial muscles?
- Arms: are they unable to lift their arms, or do they have weakness or numbness in one or other of them?
- Speech: is the person slurring or their speech unclear?
- Take action: if someone is experiencing these symptoms, act immediately and call 999.

Some of these symptoms might mean someone has had a mini-stroke (sometimes known as a 'warning stroke'), and helping them quickly can stop them from having a more serious stroke in the future. If you have had a mini-stroke (or Transient Ischaemic Attack, a TIA) in the past, changing your lifestyle and taking prescribed medication will help with managing your condition.

Many of the lifestyle factors that prevent high blood pressure and diabetes and so on also help reduce the likelihood of you having a stroke in the future. Shall I remind you of them again? Eating healthily and staying active, not smoking and cutting down alcohol.

Managing life after a stroke can be frustrating, and there are resources available to help. Your rehabilitation team in hospital will consist of specialist nurses, occupational therapists and physiotherapists. They can all help you regain your strength, stamina and independence. The Stroke Association also runs local support groups to provide emotional and physical support.

Musculoskeletal conditions

Bone or joint pain affects most people at some point in their lives, but for one in four of us, musculoskeletal conditions (MSK), such as arthritis, back pain, osteoporosis and over 200 other conditions, are a more permanent feature. Although they have a mix of symptoms and treatments, almost all MSK conditions affect older people the most, and can really have an impact on your quality of life.

Things such as keeping weight down and exercising can sometimes reduce your chance of developing MSK but preventing bone weakness associated with age can be difficult. Seventy per cent of people over 70 have arthritis in at least one part of their body. But it's possible to reduce inflammation and flare-ups with gentle exercises and strengthening activities. Of course, staying healthy can make you better able to handle any age-related conditions and pain. As with most long-term health conditions, there's a genetic component to MSK as well, and there are known links between certain health behaviours and types of MSK; smoking increases your likelihood of developing rheumatoid arthritis, for example.

There are many ways in which pain can be managed and damage to your joints and bones limited. Hydrotherapy, and other gentle exercises in water, can improve mobility and joint stiffness. Physical and occupational therapy can help you design a personalised programme of exercises specifically targeted at stretching and strengthening your joints. And even if you think it's going to be painful, or not the right thing to do, any physical activity you take part in will help increase mobility in your joints and bones and strengthen your muscles – talk to your GP or physio about the best way to do this.

NHS England provides a comprehensive range of resources for all MSK conditions. And Versus Arthritis, which provides support for the 10 million people with arthritis, are also doing research on the early detection of autoimmune disorders and other factors that can prevent significant joint and bone damage.

The less recognised or talked about pillar of physical activity is strength and balance. Having muscle strength, good bone density and the ability to balance is absolutely crucial as you get older, not only to prevent and manage musculoskeletal conditions like arthritis, but also to reduce your risk of a fall and keep you independent for longer. With a good ability to grip, and to get up out of your chair, support your body as you bathe and go to the loo, you'll be able to stay independent all your life. People struggle to imagine what it might be like not to be able to do these things and so don't take protective action to keep themselves strong and mobile now. But the Chief Medical Officer's advice for adults is specifically to do three things – do 30 minutes of moderate aerobic exercise a day, have less sedentary time, and do two sessions of strength and balance a week. These don't have to be gym based – walk up the stairs 20 times a day, carry shopping home, do heavy gardening or DIY. Stand on one leg for 30 seconds while brushing your teeth! There are plenty of activities that you can build in; Dr Muir Gray's excellent book with Diana Moran (the Green Goddess), *Sod Sitting Get Moving!*, gives wonderfully illustrated advice for how to improve your strength and balance among other ways to keep physically active.

Some people are gym bunnies. For others, the environment is intimidating and the cost off-putting. But there might be an outdoor gym near you. With specially designed equipment to help enhance balance and strength skills, these outdoor facilities are easy to use and completely free. There are lots of these around the country – your local authority website should have details.

And for those who want an easy way into running, parkrun is a great way to start. Parkrun does what you might imagine – organises local 5km runs every Saturday morning. They're free and for all ages and abilities – you just need to register once. Nearly 1.9 million people have already joined the scheme, and you don't need to go with the aim of breaking the running records – many people walk the distance, or you could jog with friends, or indeed volunteer to help organise runs.

Chronic Obstructive Pulmonary Disease (COPD)

Chronic Obstructive Pulmonary Disease (COPD) is an umbrella term used to describe progressive lung diseases including emphysema, chronic bronchitis and refractory (non-reversible) asthma. This condition is characterised by increasing breathlessness.

Perhaps unsurprisingly, the biggest risk factor in the development of COPD is smoking. Some cases are caused by industrial conditions or genetic predisposition, but smoking is now the biggest factor in getting it. So, if you haven't heard this enough so far, here it is again: please stop smoking!

Sometimes, working around harmful fumes or dust can cause damage or scarring to the lining of your lungs, and lead to the development of COPD years later. It's true of course that fewer people now work in industries (like mining or being exposed to asbestos) where this is likely to happen, but there is still a group of people with COPD who developed it while working in those industries. Repeated breathlessness and persistent coughing are not 'just a sign you're getting older' – they could indicate problems with your lungs.

You can't fully reverse damage already caused to your lungs, but there are many ways to reduce symptoms and allow you to get on with your life. Maintaining a healthy weight is vital, as being over- or underweight can make your symptoms worse. Keeping fit and doing regular exercise can also help. Like MSK and worrying about pain that exercise might cause, it might feel counterintuitive to do exercise that leads to breathlessness, but the breathlessness that comes with exercising will reduce with time and, in fact, inactivity will *increase* episodes of breathlessness.

The British Lung Foundation has a lot of information on exercises you can practise to increase lung capacity and cope with coughing episodes or breathlessness. As with asthma, inhalers and medications such as corticosteroids might be prescribed for you. Pulmonary rehabilitation, a system of physical exercises and COPD education, is also sometimes used by healthcare teams to help manage the condition.

The bottom line is that in most cases, COPD is preventable, and the best preventive action is to stop smoking. Your GP can help you access support groups and offer advice on how to stop smoking for good.

Dementia

Dementia is an umbrella term used to describe a myriad of diseases of the brain, mainly associated with symptoms like decline in memory or other thinking skills severe enough to reduce someone's ability to perform everyday activities. The most prevalent dementia type is Alzheimer's disease, accounting for 60–80 per cent of cases, but there are others including vascular dementia, Lewy body dementia, Parkinson's disease dementia, and CJD.

As of 2015, there were 850,000 people in the UK living with some form of dementia, more than 800,000 of whom are over 65. By 2040, this will be over 1.2 million.

Managing the symptoms of dementia can be difficult, and both the Alzheimer's Society and Dementia UK provide great resources for people with dementia, their carers and others. They can provide practical help and are also carrying out research on how to prevent dementia or delay the onset of symptoms after diagnosis.

The Dementia Friends movement has five simple messages for you to remember and act on, to better understand and help those who have the condition:

1. Dementia is not a natural part of ageing and is not going to happen to everyone. Some young people get it, and many older people don't.
2. Dementia is an illness like any other. It is caused by different diseases of the brain. Like any disease, your likelihood of developing it varies based on family history, your lifestyle and chance.

3. Changes in memory are not the only symptoms of dementia. It can also affect behaviour, co-ordination and sight among other things. However, short-term memory loss is often one of the first symptoms that people notice in their loved ones.
4. It is possible to live well with dementia! There is still a life to live, and people with the condition shouldn't be labelled 'sufferers'. They can still enjoy spending time with friends and family, learn new things and have happy times.
5. Dementia does not define a person, and people with the disease are more than just a collection of their symptoms. You wouldn't define a person with diabetes as only a 'diabetic' – you should make sure you see beyond the dementia to the person.

Contrary to popular belief, there are steps you can take to prevent some kinds of dementia – particularly vascular dementia. According to Dementia UK, 'what's good for the heart is good for the brain'. So – recognising a pattern here? – reduce alcohol and stop smoking, adopt a healthy diet and an active lifestyle.

Prevent dementia by speaking Swahili

There are some other surprising – and maybe even enjoyable – preventive actions you could take. Research shows that learning and practising a language has a protective effect on the brain and works to keep it healthy. Dr Thomas Bak, a Reader in Human Cognitive Neuroscience at the University of Edinburgh, is an expert in the effect of language learning on the brain, and I asked him about the link between languages and brain health:

'I worked for 20 years with dementia patients and found that learning a new language has a protective effect and can help delay symptoms. Practically, there's nothing stopping you from learning a language in later life – and you see improvement in cognitive health even after a week of learning. But it's not just about learning – you have to practise too. Knowing how to swim and not actually swimming won't improve your health, and mental exercise is similar to physical exercise.

'Learning a new language is one of the best ways to do this. You learn new sounds, rules, concepts, and even different social rules, like the difference between "vous" and "tu" in French. And if you learn in a group, there's the added positive effect of social interaction. When you practise a lot, and if you know more than one language, when looking at objects – let's say there's a squirrel in the garden, you "see" all the possible ways of naming the creature. *Squirrel* in English. *Ardilla* in Spanish. *Ecureuil* in French. You have an activation and selection going on, sometimes consciously, sometimes automatically.

'We don't know exactly how it works to keep us mentally healthy – it's easy to measure blood pressure going down if you do more exercise, and how physical activity keeps us healthy. Not so easy with the brain. But we think it's likely to work through increasing synaptic density, potentially increasing the amount of white matter and connections in the brain. And the more of this you have – your "cognitive reserve" – the healthier your brain is, for longer.

'I would recommend searching online for *Lingo Flamingo* – a great resource for learning and helping prevent and manage dementia.'

Of course, learning a language isn't the only activity that can help with brain health. One study compared the cognitive health of two groups of people, one that spent time every week doing non-demanding tasks, such as watching a film or socialising, and the other learning digital photography or quilting. Unsurprisingly, the group learning a new skill had better cognitive ability.

Dr Bak speaks seven languages – impressive. He said that while lots of practice – up to five hours a week – shows an amazing improvement on brain health, similarly to physical activity, even small amounts help. So perhaps now's the time to dust off those language learning CDs (or borrow some from the library), join a local conversation group, or start a course in Spanish, Japanese or Swahili!

Mental health

Having good mental health is just as important as avoiding or managing physical disease, and we've seen a welcome movement to talk and understand more about mental health over the last few years, as well as prevent poor mental health where possible and treat it on a par with physical health. But the extent of poor mental health in older people is shockingly high and feels hidden in wider society.

- Twenty-two per cent of men and 28 per cent of women over 65 are thought to suffer from clinical depression. But only 25 per cent of these receive treatment for their conditions.
- It's estimated that up to 40 per cent of older adults in full-time care suffer from depressive disorders, and these often go unnoticed.
- Some of the most common triggers for depression include retirement, bereavement, being on your own and disability. These factors often affect people as they age and dealing with them can be difficult.

Have you seen any of these symptoms in someone you know?

- Turning down invitations or social events that they'd usually enjoy.
- Not seeming to get much happiness out of visits.
- Neglecting their appearance or personal hygiene.
- Complaining of feeling worthless.

Nearly 8 million people over 55 experience depression, and 7 million have anxiety. But don't despair. There is support for you, or someone you care about, to help improve mental health. Try and speak to a healthcare professional. Your GP can advise on your condition and talking your fears through may help. If you just want to learn more, you can visit the government's website dedicated to helping improve older adults' mental health, MindEd.

Eyes, ears, feet and other bits

As well as long-term conditions like COPD, and serious 'events' like cancer and stroke, there are some common problems faced by older adults (and many people in 'middle age'). If they begin to affect ageing relatives, or yourself, there are ways to manage and get help.

Foot Problems

As you get older, the joints in your feet begin to wear down and the skin becomes more fragile. This can cause pain, discomfort, and sometimes bunions. Toenails may also start to claw. This might not apply to you yet (or ever!) – but perhaps for older parents or friends, here's some advice on what to do about it:

- The old favourite: exercise. It builds strength and flexibility in your feet and improves balance.
- It's really important to wear the right footwear. Slippers can encourage a 'shuffle', whereas something with a supported arch and straps keeping your feet firmly in place is better for your feet and won't draw stares when you're at the shops in the way slippers might!
- If you have a pre-existing long-term condition, particularly diabetes, make sure to keep an eye out for any changes, cuts and sores in your feet and see your GP if you spot anything.
- If you have a health condition, you can ask your GP to be referred to an NHS podiatrist if you're having trouble with foot health and maintenance. If you're housebound, they might come to your home.

Hearing Problems

It's the ultimate caricature of 'old age' – sitting in a bath chair with an ear trumpet at the ready. And yes, it's true that 4 in 10 people over the age of 50 do have some level of hearing loss. But, as with other conditions, there's lots to be done, and it doesn't need to stop you or any older people you know having a good life. Hearing loss is usually gradual, and you might not even notice it until it's pointed out to you. It's really important to do something about this; the sooner you deal with it, the better equipped you will be to carry on as normal. Pretending your hearing isn't going (and living up to the stereotype of turning up the TV ever LOUDER) isn't great for you, your family, friends or other folk. Your GP might refer you to an Ear, Nose and Throat (ENT) specialist at the hospital, and you should be entitled to a free NHS hearing aid, if you want it. Most NHS hearing aids are the traditional behind the ear kind, and NHS lists can sometimes involve a wait, but if you're looking for something more discreet, you can get ones that fit inside your ear canal and are hardly visible. Some high street retailers have monthly plans to spread out payments for hearing aids and the cost of follow-up care, batteries and repairs. Of course, you might choose to go for a private assessment instead. How you adapt to your changing hearing is up to you, and you don't need to buy expensive equipment if it's not right for you. The national charity Action on Hearing Loss has lots of information on what to expect, and resources to help you.

Vision Problems
Having issues with sight is also very common. It's really important to get annual eye checks when you're over the age of 40 because severe sight loss may, in fact, be preventable.

- Get regular eye checks, and go back if there are any changes in your vision.
- Know your family history, especially if it includes diabetes or glaucoma, where the optic nerve becomes damaged and sight loss can occur.

- The mantra: eat healthily and exercise. Long-term conditions that develop as a result of poor diet and lack of exercise, like diabetes, can be seriously harmful to your eye health.
- Stop smoking. (You probably don't, right? But just in case you do…) Smoking is proven to correlate strongly with the development of glaucoma in later life.

You can find further resources on the website for the Royal National Institute of Blind People, who cover all aspects of sight loss.

Continence

And now, the 'butt' of all jokes about old age – incontinence. It might be funny to some, but it can actually lead to social withdrawal and have a negative impact on mental health. Lots of health problems can lead to incontinence, from urinary tract infections and prostate problems to Alzheimer's disease and age-related muscle weakness. It's not easy, or indeed always possible, to prevent incontinence in older men and women, but it can be managed so that you can lead a normal life.

- It's important to find the cause of the problem. It's is not necessarily a natural part of ageing, and an inability to control your bladder may be down to something like a urinary tract infection – easy to pick up and eminently treatable.
- You can do exercises to help strengthen the bladder and bowel. Your GP can advise you on the ones most suitable for you.
- There are lots of products designed to help deal with incontinence, like disposable bedding, pads and bed protectors. You might qualify to receive these free on the NHS, but they can also be bought in pharmacies.

Given how widespread incontinence is, let's be proactive, deal with it, and perhaps even talk about it more? Reducing the stigma about this and other frequently experienced bodily changes in later life would be good for all of us.

Menopause

Here's a quiz question for you. What do half the population on average experience for four years of their middle age, and can have symptoms including night sweats, hot flushes, vaginal dryness, loss of sex drive, difficulty sleeping, feeling depressed or anxious, problems with memory and concentration, and recurrent urinary tract infections; and yet is hardly ever mentioned? Yes – hopefully you have guessed it (or indeed may be going through it) – the menopause. Why don't we talk more about it, bar the raging debate about HRT, which is still officially advised as a treatment to relieve symptoms? You may have a view on the taboo. Some people are trying to break the taboo and reduce the stigma, including Menopause Matters UK, which publishes blogs, posts information on a website and regularly appears in the media, and the Menopause Café movement, with meetings springing up all over Britain.

Diet

Most people over 65 have the same diet as everyone else but that often changes when they get older – at around age 75. And diet can deteriorate a lot when people get into extreme old age. The reasons for this are complex, and can be a mix of medical, psychological and physical factors. Loneliness will often play a part, if the partner of an older person has passed away. This could be something you recognise as a risk for yourself, but you might be thinking of an older relative here – if you think that this is happening, what can you do? It's always a good idea to get them to talk to their GP; maybe go with them if you can. It is hard, though, to knit together the services your older friend/relative may need and you may need to help navigate the system to get the right support. If you're discussing diet, or providing food for them, recognise that even if your relative/friend is very old and frail, nutritional advice still applies. Look for ways to add fat and calories if they are underweight – one cannot live off tea and biscuits alone! Lunch clubs might work if social isolation might be part of the problem, and think about the social element of eating – including factors like transport if you invite them round for dinner. But while it's tempting to give people menu advice, psychological factors like loneliness, as mentioned, or depression could be an underlying factor. Badly fitting dentures, arthritis affecting the ability to use a knife or open jars, and medication affecting the taste or appetite could be reasons for not eating. Be a bit of a detective but try not to tell people what to do. Oh – and a vitamin D supplement is a good idea for when you're older. It can be difficult to get enough Vitamin D from diet, and it not only keeps bones strong but helps with wider physical and mental health.

NHS – Healthy Diet Plate

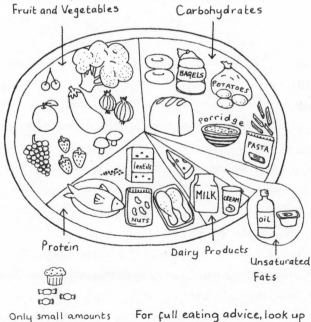

Fruit and Vegetables

Carbohydrates

Protein

Dairy Products

Unsaturated Fats

Only small amounts of sugary snacks

For full eating advice, look up the Eatwell guide online

Getting heavy

In every section about how to prevent and manage disease or illness so far, you will have noticed – in fact, you won't have been able to miss it – that your eating habits play a huge part in your health. So just a few more words about the weighty subject of obesity before moving on. I talked to Dr Alison Tedstone, who is the Chief Nutritionist at Public Health England, and asked her to paint the picture of how the population has changed in its eating habits, and the impact this has had on almost all of us.

'On average, diets in the UK are pretty poor. We're eating too much saturated fat, too much sugar, too much salt, too little fibre, not enough fruit and veg, and not enough oily fish. We've recently estimated how many calories people are consuming every day (by checking how much they would need to eat and drink to maintain their current weight) and found that people are simply eating and drinking too many calories. So, there are very high rates of ill health related to being overweight and obese like heart disease, many cancers and Type 2 diabetes. Over the years, our eating patterns have got worse. Historically, diets were better – our body weights have gone up over time. If we think about the environments we live in now, we have more food choice, more advertising, more opportunities to buy and eat food – and our food is cheaper in real terms. We're spending the lowest proportion of our family income on food than ever before. We've got what we want in a sense – more leisure time and plentiful cheap food. But our pattern of food consumption is simply making us unhealthy.

'People do know what they should be doing differently on the whole. Most people can give you a broad sense of what a healthy diet is. And there are things that you can do. People can help themselves by being more aware of what they're eating, putting in place goals for changing their diet (eating less, and more healthily), reading food labels, cooking from scratch and recognising that they can save money by doing this. There's rhetoric out there that healthy food is more expensive. That might be true if you buy a "healthier" pizza than an "unhealthier" one, but if you make yourself tomato sauce and pasta and a few veggies that's likely to be cheaper and better for you. The reality is, your best intentions fail you when you see four chocolate bars for a pound in the supermarket – you'd have to be superhuman to resist that. We like to think we've got free will in terms of our eating habits, but what you are buying is governed by the food industry.

'The government knows that people need to be supported in making healthier choices. That's why we've got the sugar levy on soft drinks and restrictions on food advertised to children – and more needs to be done. The mere announcement of the tax made some people sit up and understand quite how much sugar was actually in fizzy drinks. And if you now see that your choice is perhaps not as much down to your free will as you imagined, you can play a role in helping change the system as well. Make a noise about it. One of my bugbears is when you go for a swim in your council pool, the vending machines are selling more calories than you've burnt off. Write to them saying "Hey guys how about healthy vending please?". If schools are giving unhealthy food to your kids, write to school governors challenging them to do better. Go beyond complaining to your friends. Write to your council leader, your MP, your kids' school, the manager of your leisure centre. If you see a drinks company sponsoring your local football club, start a Twitter campaign!

'I hear the cries of "I am an adult, don't tell me what to do" – but poor diet is just a lose-lose situation. Not just for your own health, but because through our taxes we pay for the cost of diet-related disease – obesity costs the NHS £6 billion alone a year and wider society £23 billion.'

Changing your ways – not easy but possible

Recently, health authorities have been trying to help people to change their behaviours in small ways every day, to make themselves just a bit healthier. You might have seen the One You campaign publicity from Public Health England. Focusing on improving health from middle age onwards, their take is that modern life is 'ganging up on us' and making it hard for us to make healthy choices. By the time we reach our 40s, our habits may have already had a negative impact on our health in later life without even realising it.

The One You campaign has advice on how to fit getting and staying healthy into your busy schedule. There's the 400/600/600 rule, for example. This is about how many calories your meals should be: 400 for breakfast, 600 for lunch and dinner. If you can manage to discipline yourself and build calorie counting into your routine, it could cut inches off your waist.

And what about the oft-mentioned need to exercise more? Walking a brisk 10 minutes three times every day is a great way to get your quota in. The app Active10 can help you start and keep it up. Brisk short walks are a good way to change your daily routine. Walking to the car, sitting at a desk for eight hours and then coming home to sit on the sofa is not enough exercise for anyone, but especially not if you're in middle age. You know you do it, the work-sofa thing. Time to break the routine.

You might have heard of this great motivational tool: Couch to 5K from the NHS website. This campaign aims to get you from couch potato to certified runner, covering a significant distance in nine weeks and building your strength every day. Parkrun, mentioned earlier in the book, is also a good way to get running. You can download apps on your phone or other digital device, listen to podcasts with tips on how to use the programme and join a Facebook support group to make contact with others who are trying to move a little more.

Just a small one

Booze. Why do we love it so? We enjoy it to wind down after a hard day, have a laugh with friends, celebrate special occasions, and just because. I too like to have a drink. But, and we all do know this, there's a big difference between moderate drinking and causing yourself harm by hitting the hard stuff. The recommended maximum amounts are 14 units a week. This is set by the Chief Medical Officer, who examines the evidence for the level of risk that drinking excessively presents. Britons drink 9.5 litres of alcohol per capita per year on average. This compares to 8.6 litres in Spain and 8.8 in the USA. While there's a trend in younger generations to drink less, 55–64-year-olds are the most likely to be drinking at high and dangerous levels, especially the wealthier groups in that age range. On average, middle-aged men (45–64-year-olds) drink 37 units a week (the equivalent of 16 pints of beer). Many people do understand the link between alcohol and diseases like cancer (as well as the link between alcohol and hangovers) and are trying to cut down. An estimated 5 million people took part in 'dry January' in 2017. In fact, doctors would rather we abstain totally for two consecutive days a week at least, to give our livers time to recover. If you want to reduce the amount you drink, take small steps to help – order drinks with a lower alcohol content or get a half pint instead of a full one. Smaller wine glasses at home might help with reducing the volume. Even small changes could improve your health and reduce the risk that too much booze brings.

Are you convinced now that doing more exercise and eating more healthily – losing a few pounds, and trying to keep them off, and cutting back on the booze – could be some of the most important things you do as you get older? And yes – I *am* on a diet.

So, to sum up – pretty much everyone thinks that good health is, or will be, our biggest asset in later life, so we need to invest in it now. You can prevent getting long-term conditions, or at least delay their onset, but if and when you do get disease, or experience changes in how well you hear, see and pee, it's not the end of the world. Managing it well will mean you're still able to work if you want to and enjoy life in other ways. You will be entirely familiar with the essential guidelines by now:

1. Stay at a healthy weight;
2. Don't smoke;
3. Reduce your alcohol intake;
4. Do some physical activity, including strength and balance exercises.

Remember, your mental health is as important as your physical health, and activities outlined in other chapters including work, volunteering and being connected to others will contribute to good mental health. If you struggle with starting or keeping up healthy habits, there's lots of support and help available – and if you want to stop the food and drink pushers making it more difficult to stay on the right path, join in the campaign against junk!

7

WHERE YOU'LL LIVE

We've talked a lot about what you're going to do in later life – but where are you going to do it?! Thinking about your neighbourhood, village, town or city, do you hanker to stay put, or are you one of the millions who engage in 'property porn', stalking the perfect bungalow in Billericay, and wondering if house prices will go up or down? If you're renting now, what are your options for moving? If you own your home, is it a risk to release the equity, or savvy to trade your home in for your perfect retirement pad elsewhere? Whether you want to move or not, where you live, including how safe and connected with others you feel, and how easy it is to get around, is going to be crucial to your future health and happiness.

First, let's think about what's really important to you. On the next page is an exercise that might help you prioritise. Put a tick next to each statement you agree with, then if you think you already feel like this, put another tick under 'already have'.

If more than half of your answers have two ticks, should you think about moving at all? If all of them have double ticks, you are living in a pretty wonderful area!

Where there are no ticks in the 'already have' column – say on how safe you feel, or how walkable your neighbourhood is – and these factors are strong motivations to move home, think about whether the area you'd like to move to does have these features. Spend time visiting, look at local online forums and examine the local authority website where there's normally info on cultural, leisure and volunteering activities as well as any plans for regeneration. Police.uk

Elements of your perfect place to live	Would like to feel this	Already have!
I feel safe walking around my neighbourhood, even at night	☐	☐
I can keep healthy and active – streets are easy to walk around and there's not too much traffic. Local parks mean there's lots of green space and leisure centres have options that help me keep fit	☐	☐
There are lots of places I can meet friends and neighbours – from cafés to church halls and arts venues	☐	☐
Local transport systems are great	☐	☐
I can take part in local life easily – including volunteering if I want to	☐	☐
I like the design of buildings, streets and houses near where I live and public buildings are easy to navigate	☐	☐
I can pursue my hobbies and interests in my local area	☐	☐

has information on crime rates in every area, and there's nothing to stop you calling the local community police team for a chat about crime rates and keeping safe.

Most people actually want to stay in their own home and neighbourhood as they grow older. Perhaps it's worth thinking about whether or not the area you already love to live in could be improved and even if you might be able to help make that happen. There's a growing movement called Age-friendly Cities and Communities that aims to make all areas great for people in later life to live in.

Age-friendly communities

In 2006 the World Health Organization (WHO) launched their guide on Age-friendly Cities. Since then there's been lots of interest in this approach, which has grown internationally, leading to the development of the WHO Global Network of Age-Friendly Cities and Communities, with hundreds of cities and communities signed up worldwide. But what is an age-friendly community or city?

The WHO says there are eight major elements to somewhere being age-friendly:

1. Outdoor space and public buildings. It's common sense that when people feel safe where they live and have good local amenities, they do more outdoors. Accessible public buildings, pavement and street design are really important, particularly if you've got a disability or a condition that limits you. Attractive and walkable spaces including parks, seating and public loos can make all the difference in your local area.

2. Transport. Reliable, affordable, frequent public transport – with bus and rail routes that go where you want to go – is important anyway, but increasingly so when driving becomes stressful or challenging.

3. Housing. As mentioned right at the beginning of this book, most people want to grow old in their own homes. Having affordable housing that's adapted to your needs, in a choice of styles, types of tenure and in neighbourhoods you want to live in, is essential for age-friendly communities.

4. Participation. Being with friends, family, neighbours and meeting new people. Some people are happy spending most of their time on their own. Others love being surrounded by other folk. Most of us are probably somewhere in between, valuing time spent with friends and family, passing the time of day with neighbours and acquaintances, but also needing some 'me time'. Whatever your preference, an age-friendly area should make your choice a reality, offering opportunities to take part in community and social activities when people want them.

5. Respect! Feeling included and respected, with people in your area understanding that those in later life have a valuable role to play, is an important factor in any age-friendly community. Are there positive images of ageing on display, and a good understanding between generations to challenge negative attitudes?

6. Volunteering and paid work. An age-friendly area is one where there are opportunities to be in fulfilling work for those who want to or need to be, including flexible and part-time work. Volunteering, becoming politically active, or being part of local groups and organisations should all be options as well. All these types of activities give meaning and purpose to many (as well as the obvious financial benefits of being in paid work).

7. Communication and information. Staying in touch with friends and family, and learning about local events, news and activities are all important elements of the 'age-friendly' idea. Age-friendly communities are likely to help people get online, but also make sure that information is made available in other ways, for those who don't use the internet.

8. Accessible and affordable health and care services. This is obviously a crucial part of any local system to keep people in later life healthy, independent and active. Care and health services need to be conveniently located to where older people live, with adequately trained staff. A wide variety of services are required, including helping prevent people becoming ill or injuring themselves (e.g. through a fall) in the first place. But also, the provision of social care at home, day centres, care homes and support and respite facilities for carers needs to be excellent, as well as having end of life care.

The Centre for Ageing Better is helping co-ordinate communities that are committed to becoming more age-friendly. At the time of writing (list from August 2018), they are: Banbury, Belfast, Brighton and Hove, Bristol, Coventry, Derry, Glasgow, Greater Manchester, Isle of Wight, Leeds, Liverpool, London, London Borough of Lewisham, London Borough of Southwark, Manchester, Melksham, Middlesbrough, Newcastle upon Tyne, Nottingham, Salford, Sefton, Sheffield, Stockport, Stoke-on-Trent, Sunderland and West Cheshire.

Get involved! They really need local people to help with ideas and designing ways your local area can be better across all the areas listed above. The details of the age-friendly community co-ordinators are on our website and on the relevant council websites.

Age-friendly Isle of Wight

The Isle of Wight is one of the members of the age-friendly communities network, and the local Age UK has spearheaded initiatives to make it a great place to grow old in. Their website hosts resources and information, including, for example, how you can start your own business after 50.

As an age-friendly community, the Isle of Wight has committed to making outdoor spaces, buildings and houses age-friendly, as well as making sure that community-based services understand the needs of older service users. They've also made a commitment to ensure older people have more of a chance to participate and have their interests and needs listened to just as much as the rest of the community.

So far on the Isle of Wight, over 200 professionals, from the police to housing associations, and more than 2000 school children have taken part in age-friendly training. There's even a radio station run by, and aimed at, older people. Every first and third Wednesday of the month, 'Older and Wiser' covers a range of topics aimed at over 55s.

There's also a movement to make places 'dementia-friendly'. The Alzheimer's Society defines this as 'a city, town or village where people with dementia are understood, respected and supported, and confident they can contribute to community life. In a dementia-friendly community, people will be aware of and understand dementia, and people with dementia will feel included and involved, and have choice and control over their day-to-day lives.'

This may well become important to you. I talked about the increase in dementia in the UK and people's particular worry about it for themselves, friends and family in Chapter Six – so it's also worth checking out if where you want to live has a commitment to being dementia friendly. There's lots of useful information online at Alzheimer's UK.

So, when considering whether or not you want to stay in your own house and neighbourhood or make a move to somewhere that might suit your needs better, there's lots to think about. If you're staying put, could you help your area become more age-friendly? Moving out means planning wisely, thinking about what you really want in your local community (beautiful environment/great transport/lots to see and do/good social connections), and prioritising accordingly.

Living abroad

The age-friendly city and community movement isn't just confined to the UK – there were 720 places globally signed up in August 2018, and the World Health Organization hopes that thousands more places will make the commitment to become age-friendly.

Many people in the UK don't just think local when considering where to live in later life – they think global! Eleven thousand people over the age of 60 went to live in another country in 2017, with by far the most popular destination for a sunny later stage of life being Spain, where nearly 120,000 British pensioners were living in 2017. If a big move abroad is part of your plans, there's a lot to think about and understand in advance before you can enjoy the sun, sand and sangria in a carefree fashion.

Here's a taste of some of the areas you'd need to consider before moving. You have to register with the Spanish Government and get a residence certificate, which includes an NIE (foreigners identification number) – essential for getting a bank account, owning property and running a car, among other things. Healthcare in Spain is different to the UK and your right to free healthcare depends on whether or not you pay social security contributions in Spain and other factors – the healthcareinspain.eu website gives more details. Gov.uk also has heaps of information on tax matters, employment, driving, voting, buying property, and what happens if you want to return to the UK. So be prepared. You'll need to think about local healthcare systems, property laws, your legal status as a resident, portability of UK state pensions and benefits, whether you can vote in elections in the UK or your new home country, and crucially, what might happen if you want to return to the UK. This is true of any country you choose, whether or not it's in Europe. And obviously all of this is also subject to change depending on the developing situation of Britain's relationship with the European Union. The key thing to remember if considering a move abroad is to research and prepare in great detail before you go.

Oh and by the way, it's always a good idea to learn the language of the country you're moving to, in case your living needs stretch further than 'dos cervezas, por favor'!

Living in the UK

Back in the UK, while we know that most people want to stay in the house and neighbourhood they're familiar with, there are an increasing number of over 55s moving to a new home every year. The English Housing Survey, which began gathering data in 2008, shows that around 280,000 households over 55 reported moving home in 2016. There's been a small but steady rise in the percentage of people over 55 moving, from just over 2 per cent in 2009 to nearly 4 per cent in 2016. (We're good at measuring things in Britain, aren't we?!)

Getting around

Once you've sorted out the kind of house you want to be in and some broad principles about the kind of neighbourhood, village, town or city you would like to be your own, it's time to think about getting around. You'll want to be able to get to your friends, family, grandkids, allotment, shops, darts club, yoga group, church, pub quiz nights, and airport for your frequent trips to Miami (insert your list here!).

Try thinking of a '20-minute rule' when thinking about moving. What can you get to within a 20-minute walk, and a 20-minute drive (whether you're driving yourself, or taking lifts, taxis or public transport)? Planners in the USA have started to think about the idea of a '20-minute village' when looking at local services located a reasonable distance from where you live – this could be a good guide for town planners here.

The phrase 'the 20-minute village' was made popular by Gerding Edlen, an urban development company based in Oregon. They believed that less time spent on travel 'means more time for family and friends, leisure activities and other meaningful experiences'. According to them, the ideal is 20 minutes on foot, but 20 minutes by public transport, bike or even by car would be a reasonable goal. You might think that walking a mile to get a pint of milk could stretch the concept a bit (unless you've taken the advice about walking more!) – so 'hamlets' or at least a few services within five minutes' walk of where you live would be a boon, with a more substantial high street 20 minutes away.

In the USA, these kinds of communities are also showing a rise in property prices, with walkability being a draw for buyers. And while the '20-minute village' can happen by happy accident, particularly if you live in a big city, it can also happen by design. Portland in Oregon, for example, is planning for 90 per cent of its neighbourhoods to be 20-minute villages by 2030. Could it be possible in the UK to create more neighbourhoods, towns and villages where this is the case? Better transport, more thought in planning services, and encouraging a good mix of shops and amenities would all be possible with the help of local authorities.

Age-friendly cities and communities across the UK consider planning and services through the lens of our ageing population, but many areas are perhaps less easy to live in for older people. As an individual thinking where to live as you age, the '20-minute village' idea could be food for thought when you make your choice. A 20-minute walk will of course also contribute towards the 30 minutes of brisk walking you'll be doing as part of your new exercise regime!

Let's think about your future mobility; depending on how well you can get around now, how long will you be able to maintain this for? If you are fit and able to walk good distances now, there's no reason why you shouldn't do this all the way through to your 'old' old age. Over time, some people might find this difficult to maintain so a 'plan B' will be useful when thinking about how to get around.

For yourself, friends or family who are older, more needs to be done to make local areas walkable. It's probably no surprise to anyone over the age of 65 to find that traffic lights really don't give you enough time to cross the road safely. One study has shown that more than three-quarters of people over 65 walk slower than the pace needed to cross in time. All in all, we need a revamp of our built environment so that everyone can fully enjoy being out and about outside as they age.

Keep on trucking!

Do you drive now? If you do, great – but in the future you might not want to drive long distances to get to your local amenities. Most people who drive now will want to carry on doing so, and it's a real wrench if you have to stop. The law says that you have to reapply for your licence at 70 and then get checked every three years after that.

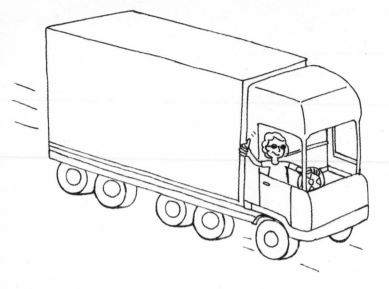

If your eyesight (with glasses) and reflexes and general health are fine, then all should be well. You can take refresher courses – as your reflexes slow down, and perhaps your range of neck movement changes, you might modify your decision-making a little when you're driving. Refresher courses and lessons for older drivers are provided by the Royal Society for the Prevention of Accidents, private driving companies, and in some areas your local authority. Drivers over 70 in Herefordshire can take a refresher course in driving for just £10, for example. Find out what's going to be able to help you and take action to keep driving as long as possible. And ignore the ageist media reports about 'pensioners driving the wrong way down dual carriageways' – there's no safe or unsafe age for a driver. By 2035 there will be 21 million 'older drivers' on UK roads. Currently, drivers over 60 have fewer crashes than younger age groups. While over 70s were involved in just over 6 per cent of road traffic accidents in 2016, those in the 25–29 age group had an accident rate nearly double this.

Some tips from the AA:

- You must tell the DVLA about any medical conditions that will affect your driving. Your GP may say when you need to do this, but it's a good idea to ask, 'Will this affect my driving?' whenever a new condition is diagnosed, or treatment given. Dementia can pose particular problems.

- You must also make sure you meet the eyesight requirement – regular eye tests will help.

- Reapplying for your licence. Once over 70 you'll have to reapply for your licence every three years. There's no test or medical, but you do have to make a medical declaration that may lead to DVLA making further investigations.

- The right car can help a lot. Larger mirrors and bigger windows help all-round vision while bigger doors and higher seats can all help getting in and out.

- If you've got a licence and are fit to drive, keep driving. Try not to become over-dependent on your partner's driving because as traffic conditions change it can be hard to take up driving again after several years off. Try to stay in practice on the roads you frequently use.

- If you're worried about your own or someone else's driving, check with neighbours or friends. Do they feel safe in the car? Would they take a lift? Do you or the other driver seem in control when reversing or manoeuvring?

- In some areas there are local authority schemes that use driving instructors to assess older drivers, but make sure this is in the sort of conditions and on the sort of roads you/they normally use.

If you have a physical disability, the Motability charity and Motability scheme might be able to help. The charity awards grants for wheelchair accessible vehicles, driving lessons for disabled people, and advance payments for lease vehicles and adaptations. If you receive mobility allowance the scheme could help you lease a new car, scooter or powered wheelchair.

If you have reduced mobility and need help getting around, you can ask your GP or another health professional to refer you to NHS Wheelchair Services. There's often a long waiting list for this, though. It includes an assessment of your mobility needs and help to keep you staying mobile. Local services vary widely so you may not be eligible for a wheelchair on the NHS; if you can afford it you can buy one privately (sometimes local authorities will give you a voucher for the portion of cost they would have covered if you get a more expensive one than they would have provided). If you can't afford to buy one yourself and aren't eligible on the NHS, you may be able to get help from a charity – look on the Better Mobility website for more details.

Buses and trains

So, what will it be like living where you want to if you're not driving any more (or didn't drive in the first place)? Here are some key things to think about:

- Will you be able to walk to the shops?
- If you don't have a car, how will you be able to bring shopping back? Will you be able to rely on lifts from friends and family?
- Will you need to use taxis, and how affordable might that be?
- Is there a bus service? How regular is it? If there isn't one – perhaps if you live in or have settled in a rural area with poor transport links – will you campaign for a decent bus route around the village?

Nine hundred and twenty-nine million bus journeys were made by older people and those with disabilities travelling at concessionary rates in England in 2016/17. But many people don't have bus routes near where they live that suit them. If you're not happy with the bus service where you live now or where you want to move to, talk to your local town or parish council. There might be a transport group that includes other people who want to improve local services. If you're having problems, other people will be too. There'll be someone elected in your local council who is in charge of transport plans – normally it's clear who they are on your council website, or if you ask at the council information desk. Give them a call! You could start to explain exactly what your situation is and what you'd like to see change. Even ask them how you could help them make that change...

Electric dreams

You're probably aware of driverless cars, but did you know there's also an accessible version of a driverless 'bus' for people with disabilities? 'Olli', an electric driverless vehicle with space for a group of people, was created by Local Motors and IBM, and is in small-scale use in some places in the USA. Olli has been designed to be as accessible as possible – it can pick up whether a person needs a wheelchair ramp, or whether someone with dementia needs reminding to get off at their stop. Olli can use cameras to read sign language and send a response to your phone. There won't be Ollies on every street corner in the UK any time soon, but it could be the minibus of the future.

We don't live in an ideal world, and a lot needs to change in our transport network to improve the way we get around. Imagine this utopian scenario: Your car has seats that swivel round so that you can sit in them and swing back into the vehicle – so you don't have to bend double to get in through the door. And then when you stop driving you have community transport that's easy to get on and off with helpful drivers or conductors. You get picked up and dropped off at a transport interchange, so you can create a seamless journey to where you want or need to go. One ticket is right for all journeys you make, and pricing structures are transparent to understand and good value. Streets are walkable, with green space, seating, public toilets, and crossings that give you enough time to get over the road. Where is this Nirvana? Like George Orwell's perfect pub, *The Moon Under Water*, unfortunately it doesn't exist. But some countries and cities are trying out ideas that could make at least part of this a reality. In Bogotá and Paris, some main streets in the city centre are pedestrianised on Sundays so people can stroll without the traffic, and in Finland, they're trialling an app that adapts the road crossing time depending on our walking speed. Moves are afoot in the UK to introduce new ways of getting around as part of the Government's Industrial Strategy 'Grand Challenge' on ageing and mobility. And as noted above, if you're fuming about the state of your local transport system and want to have a say, there are activist groups nationally (like the Campaign for Better Transport) and in some local areas.

Walking and cycling

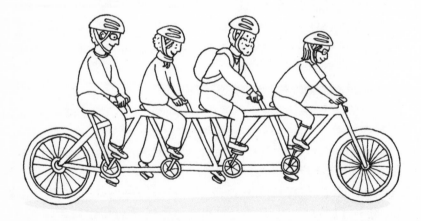

Now might be a good time to think about other kinds of transport so you're not so reliant on your car or the local bus system in later years. Take cycling up now and there's no reason why you should ever stop – it can also be a great way to meet people, perhaps by joining your local cycling group. There are national cycling clubs, listed on the Cycling UK website, and information on walking is provided by Walking for Health. Many local areas also have routes to walk and cycle on. Transport for London have introduced 'quiet routes', for example; and the Canals and River Trust has a map of the canal and river network and is working on a cycling-friendly towpath map.

You may be one of those people who prefers to ride alone, but there are some new schemes that support people to get into cycling. In Newcastle, for example, the City Council and Active Newcastle have been running training for people over 50 who've never been on a bike or want to get back on the saddle after a long period of not cycling. They have free courses, run by experts. Age UK Dudley runs weekly cycling events for over-50s, and there are many more similar schemes around the country.

Cycling for exercise or to get around is a great idea. If you want to add the option of giving your legs a rest, electric bikes are becoming very popular for people in later life.

Top five transport tips to remember:

1. Use the '20-minute rule'. Does where you want to live have the essentials of what you need within 20 minutes of walking, and a wider choice within a 20-minute drive/bus journey?

2. If you drive now, stay driving for as long as you can safely. The right car, refresher courses, and keeping mobile will all help with this.

3. If you don't drive now, or when you need to stop driving, think about all the other options – car share, community transport schemes, and the Motability scheme if appropriate for you.

4. If public transport isn't great in your chosen area, campaign to make it better! Local and national groups will be able to help with this.

5. When all else fails – walking and other self-powered options like cycling are hugely beneficial for your health.

We might take it for granted that we want to stay in the same city, town or area for the rest of our lives, or we might hanker after a major change: to be closer to the centre of town; to be in deepest rural greenery; to be closer to family or be closer to the sun and move abroad! Staying or moving, there's plenty to consider about what's going to be right for you in later life. Your ability to get around will be crucial to being connected to others as well as doing shopping and leisure activities, and as we've seen, both continuing to drive and navigating patchy public and community transport could all become challenging unless you plan, adapt and even campaign for improvement.

A great way of making a choice about where to live or improving your current neighbourhood is to look at the Age-Friendly Cities and Communities movement and help them with your views and creative ways to make change happen. Our website (ageing-better. org) has information about age-friendly cities and, if you're in or near one, how to get in touch.

8

WHAT YOUR HOME SHOULD LOOK LIKE

We're a little bit obsessed with our houses in Britain, aren't we? We're worried about how we can get on, stay on and 'climb up' the housing ladder. We think about the affordability of flats or houses in the areas of the country we'd ideally like to live, and perhaps have a fantasy of moving to the countryside, to a cottage with roses round the door, when we're in the last, pleasantly retired, part of our lives. Then the vision blurs a bit – will we have to sell our homes to pay for care, and perhaps end our lives in a council care home? Will we have to 'downsize' because we become too infirm to use the stairs or get in and out of the bath? And if we have to get a smaller place, will it suit us, and where should it be? Then the denial kicks in and we return to our vision of the fantasy cottage, quietly laying aside the mentally troublesome question of 'what then?'

So how can we best achieve our vision about where we'll live, which becomes so fundamental to our happiness and health in later life? As 6 per cent of people 65 and over – more than 600,000 people – leave their homes less than once a week, it's worth thinking about how well your home will be adapted for your later years now.

Change it up

The vast majority of us, 80 per cent, say they want to stay in their own home rather than move as they get older. People want the comfort of surroundings they're used to, to have their things around them, and to be in a community they know well. It's lovely to have mementos as well as all the other treasured possessions you've collected over the years to hand (though I'll talk about when this gets out of control – the danger of clutter and hoarding – later). Fundamentally, when we get to mid-life, most of us are settled, or at least want to stay in the home we love for as long as possible. How can we help make that a reality?

It's a case of thinking differently. Most people assume the need to change a home happens to other people, not themselves. And we often talk about home adaptations for people in later life – but the word 'adaptations' itself is problematic. It's strongly linked to disability. As well as this, if you don't have challenges moving round your home now, it's difficult to imagine what your needs might be or what that might entail in the future.

Think about the things that you do at home at the moment – the rooms you use most, what you use them for, and what your preferences are.

- How do you use your kitchen? Do you cook every day? Do you have people round for dinner and entertain much?
- Do you prefer a bath or shower, and where is the bathroom in your house?
- Have you got stairs, and if so, more than two storeys? Do you have a loft you use for storage?
- Do you have outside space and spend a lot of time there to garden or sit out in the summer?

All your preferences and the way you live now will be factors in how you might want to choose or redesign your house in the future. A lot of the principles we'll look at in terms of adapting your home might be considered 'universal design' – beautifully functional at any age. Think about this now, and particularly if you're moving. Many people will only start to think about changes once they've got a problem rather than taking an approach that builds in good design in case something happens that limits your mobility, for example.

So, people don't talk about adapting their homes much, and it's hard to know where to go to for advice. But for you or an older friend or relative, talking to an occupational therapist could be a good call, particularly when a need arises.

Let's hear some advice from occupational therapist with the OT service Kate Sheehan:

'Let me tell you about what an Occupational Therapist can do – as an OT I can help you maintain your abilities to do what you want to do, have to do, and need to do! We can look at the technique for how you go to the loo and manage your continence. We can think about how to maintain leisure activities like gardening. It's about doing your activities differently, not stopping doing them at all. OTs help you as an individual and help modify the environment you're in – for most people that's their workplace, or their home.

'I'm constantly talking to people about future-proofing their home and thinking about what a new home could look like if they're considering moving. If you might move to a new property, from age 50 onwards say, think about long-term needs. Apart from how handy the location is, will the property you're buying be able to age with you? You might be looking at refurbishments if you're moving:

'In a new **bathroom**, you might want to have a bath, but it's worth designing a shower outlet underneath it for when you might want to remove that bath and, say, have a wet room/walk in shower instead. Think about new products – new designs for digital showers that will be easier than small knobs for adjusting temperature and water flow are coming on to the market. Some new showers allow you to switch the unit on outside the shower area, so you don't have scalding or freezing water to start with. Look at the heights of toilets. For most of us, as we age our big muscles become weaker; having a slightly higher toilet will make it easier and actually more comfortable to use. Sit on them in bathroom showrooms to test them out! And if you're not moving, you can get seats that heighten the toilet. One of the key things we neglect hugely is lighting. As we age, our vision deteriorates, so you need a combination of central lighting and task lighting – especially in the bathroom for shaving, putting on make-up and so on. In England, we tend to just have one central light in the bathroom that can make those fiddly tasks difficult to achieve if you can't see well. Get a bright mirror light installed. There's nothing wrong with riser bars to help in the bath or shower – and fit a grab rail instead of a towel rail. You can get really beautiful ones now that are chrome, wooden or bespoke. They can be integrated into your bathroom without it looking medicalised. Aesthetics are changing – perhaps go to a mainstream bathroom company rather than a specialist dealer.

'In **bedrooms**, have a bed that allows you to get in and out of bed easily. More and more, I have seen people struggle with big heavy duvets. New wool duvets are very lightweight but very warm. If you have arthritis in your hands these could be much easier to handle. Lights in your room that don't have tiny switches but are voice or touch operated could also make life lots easier.

'In the **kitchen**, think about what you're going to do about placing items. Drawers instead of cupboards will be easier – and you can put internal lighting in them. If you have an oven under a counter you're bending down and lifting out hot and heavy items, so get one at eye-level if possible, plus get one with telescopic shelves that pull out and don't drop. If you're having kitchen high-level units, fit them slightly lower so you don't have to use steps or climb on anything to reach them.

'And look at your **furniture** – deep sofas and very squishy cushions might be harder to get out of when you're older. It doesn't need to be ugly! There are some beautiful pieces out there, like the 70s' Danish-style chairs and sofas with wooden arms that are becoming fashionable again now.

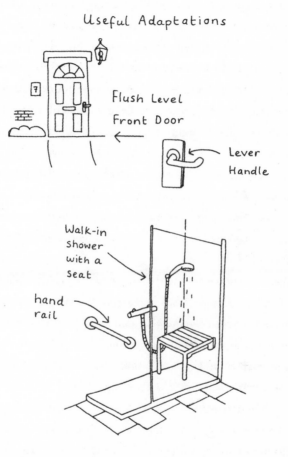

Useful Adaptations

Flush Level
Front Door

Lever
Handle

Walk-in
shower
with a
seat

hand
rail

'**Stairs** are an issue. Use them for as long as you can – they're great for maintaining your strength and balance. But when you really can't make it up or down safely, don't leave your stairlift to the last moment – it's not an end of life product. They can be really useful. I have had a client who had shortness of breath and had an office upstairs in his house. Fitting a stairlift meant he could carry on working easily. He also told me that if he hadn't had a stairlift he wouldn't have been able to sleep with his wife – you can't put a price on the ability to do that! If you think they've got some stigma about them, lose it. Stairlifts are an enabler, not a disabler.

'When you're buying **any new products** – a new fire, or an oven – check the knobs. Often they require a push and turn, which can be difficult. Insist you try before buying or make sure that the returns policy works for you.

'Change your property if necessary so it has an **entrance** with no steps, so there's no trip hazard when walking in with bags or if you start using a wheeled shopping bag. Just because you're older it doesn't mean you can't use technology – there are some excellent systems around that can be attached to doorbells so you can see who's at the front door without opening it; many of these systems can also take a picture of who's been to your house – useful for security if you're not there.

'These are all small but could be really important things. We also need natural light in our houses. If you don't have good natural lighting it can have a poor effect on your mental health – and that's the same for fresh air – so try and open windows when the weather's good enough and let as much light in as you can whatever the time of year.'

As well as changing your environment, remember any form of **exercise** is really important, from going to the gym to swimming, Pilates, gardening and getting a dog to make you walk every day. The need to be physically active and keep up your strength and balance is dealt with in another chapter, but as we don't live our lives in segregated chapters, thinking about where you live and your ability to get around the house is deeply linked to your physical and mental health, and how changes to each of these aspects of our life could have positive repercussions on the others. Kate told me about a lady she helped whose daughter had organised an occupational therapy visit. The lady had had a stroke and was spending all her time downstairs in her living room with a commode. She was depressed, not going out or doing anything. When asked why she wasn't going out, she said it was because she didn't feel she could wash herself properly and smelt (Kate assured me she didn't!). Putting in a stairlift and adapting the bathroom meant she could wash every day. As soon as she felt clean she went out, met friends, and effectively lived her old life. Her physical health and mental health improved to the point she was able to stop using the stairlift and walk up the stairs herself. Get help for yourself or others if you need it – it could be life-changing.

A few more tips for those in much later life:

- If you're worried about dementia or memory loss, certain colours can help or hinder. Putting a dark rug on pale flooring, for example, can be stressful and lead to perceptions of a hole or gap.
- Think about lever taps in sinks and levers instead of knobs for doors. These are helpful for everyone but can be especially good if you have arthritis.
- Getting someone to look specifically for trip hazards in the home can significantly reduce the risk of having a fall (the fire service do this in some areas of the country, but occupational therapists will also help) – they might suggest some simple changes, like having non-slip mats.
- You could also get remote-controlled heating or fireplaces. This means you'd be able to control the temperature from your phone, computer or tablet.
- A reading light might also be useful and won't strain your eyes as much as if you just had one main light.

The other 'generation rent'

While most of this chapter assumes you have your own home, rising house prices in many areas of the UK have meant an increase in older private renters. There has been a small but consistent rise in people privately renting over 65, with 117,000 more people in later life renting in 2016 than there had been in 1996. But then, people only needed to save for two years for a deposit in 1996, compared to

16 years in 2016, assuming no help from family or friends. This is set to rise even further, as nearly a quarter of those aged 35–44 are privately renting, with no guarantee that they will be able to buy homes in the future. Renting through your life is seen as normal in many other countries, especially in Switzerland, where about 50 per cent of all people rent privately, and in Germany, where renting throughout life is well established and tenants have very strong rights.

But in Britain the idea that if you don't own your own home by 40 you haven't 'made it' is still pervasive and can be pretty demeaning. We need to lose that attitude. But with accepting that renting will become more of the norm for more people in later life, significant changes will need to be made. We talked about adapting your home – but if you don't own it, is there any obligation on a landlord to do this, or allow you to? And the ever-present insecurity in private renting – both in terms of rent rises and tenure – makes life potentially less stable. Then there's also the question of financial security. So many people are depending on selling or releasing equity from their home to pay for care costs or have pension income, or to leave as an asset to their children. If you're renting, clearly these aren't options available to you and other ways of having enough funds for a good quality of later life become more important.

To top it off, the quality of private rented homes in the UK overall is not great. More than a quarter of all private rented properties don't meet the government's decent homes standard (27 per cent), meaning they lack basic amenities or sufficient heating, or both. This is a scandal. If you're renting and are concerned about the quality of your accommodation, or what you're being charged, understand your rights and how to get redress if things go wrong at Gov.uk and as ever, your local Citizens Advice branches can also help.

The Scottish government have recently made open-ended rental agreements mandatory, unless there are grounds for eviction. Landlords have to give three months' notice to increase rent, and tenants can appeal against this. No-fault evictions are no longer possible. If the landlord wants tenants to leave, they must prove they have a good reason for this, for example proof that they're going to sell the property. Notice periods also have to be much longer. If someone has lived at the property for more than six months, and is leaving through no fault of their own, landlords have to give them at least 84 days' notice.

Clutter and hoarding

Most people are not located at the extremes of a hoarding spectrum – neither being a minimalist with virtually no possessions, nor having 'hoarding disorder'. Extreme hoarding means you have so many objects and items in the house that you can't move from one room to another. This is a clinical condition; do get help for anyone you know who might have a hoarding disorder, first by gently encouraging them to see the GP, who may recommend therapy. People who have this condition are sometimes unable to move around and can't access parts of their home, including their bathroom and kitchen, and a negative cycle kicks in where their hygiene and mental health can suffer.

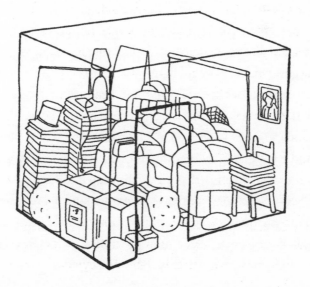

Even if you don't hoard, you may be keeping stuff unnecessarily. Some people have told me that they have found they've had to spend large amounts of time excavating the boxes, tins and magazines saved over the years from rooms and lofts after their parents die – though it can also be lovely to see and keep mementos and even antiques from parents and previous generations. My own mum was a ruthless thrower-away of things so I didn't have that particular job when she passed away! If you want to make your space more, well, spacious, try:

- Saving only the last couple of issues of magazines rather than keeping piles of back issues around.
- Have a wardrobe clear-out every year – if you haven't worn something in the last year, are you really going to wear it again?
- Donate books you're not going to read again to charity – and that goes for unloved ornaments too.
- If you move house, make a major effort to declutter *before* you go rather than when you arrive.
- Change your habits to use less to start with – the environmental movement would approve!

It's all common sense – but do dedicate time to it if you can see stuff building up around you; it will make your home feel lighter, fresher, and bigger…

Alternative housing and living

We've looked at adapting your own home, so you can stay in it for longer, and considered the trend in older private renters. As noted, less than 5 per cent of people over 65 years old are in full-time residential care, as most want to, and can, stay in their own homes. The worry is that our journey will be from home to care home or hospital (then funeral parlour?) but of course there are many other options for where to enjoy your extra years. There are at least three kinds of specialist housing for older people, including places where you have to be a certain age to be a resident, otherwise known as retirement homes or villages; or housing with or without support. Housing without support might have a warden who's around in case of problems, or a personal alarm system. Housing with support usually means that there are people who provide help with everyday tasks like bathing and taking medication.

Some purpose-built retirement communities, such as Whiteley Village in Surrey, enable older people with limited financial means and different care needs to become part of a vibrant community. The village is run by the Whiteley Homes Trust and has over 260 almshouse cottages, plus extra-care apartments and nursing care facilities. Although the Trust aims to support villagers to live at home independently for as long as possible, if their needs increase above what can be provided at home, the varied accommodation available at Whiteley means it is possible for them to move to extra care facilities if required.

Whiteley Village is part of the Almshouse Association – there are around 1600 almshouse charities, with about 35,000 properties across the country. Almshouses have historic roots in religious orders caring for the poor and have evolved into a movement to provide for those in need, often providing homes for particular groups of people like miners, fishermen and retail workers.

Dr Alison Armstrong works at Whiteley Village. She explained the model:

'We have a large collection of housing and our size means we can have extra levels of support. People often come here in their 60s or 70s, and many volunteer to help other residents. The Trust has over 100 years of data about people who've lived here, and we have found that on average people live longer at Whiteley Village. I am working with academics to research why, and we will share our findings so others can learn from our experience. Giving back to society is an important part of our charitable purpose. We have a long waiting list and would love to be able to house more people.'

And Whiteley Village resident Margaret (Peggy) Ruff told me about how wonderful it is to live there:

'Whiteley should be shared around the world. I've come here and I've never been so happy in all my life. If you want to be secluded you can and there's back up. If you want to be sociable, you can be. There's a heated swimming pool, a golf course, putting, a bowling green and billiards. We have our own post office, village shop, library and lots of clubs. There are a team of staff on site looking after all the buildings and grounds; some use special Whiteley electric vans, like the old milk vans, to get around! We live in over 200 acres, with deer, and all sorts of animal life. We've got quite a few 100-year-olds. It's wonderful. In fact, I'm positive that living here will lengthen our lives!'

While not at all common in the UK, housing co-operatives are a potential option for people who enjoy communal living. In Barnet in London, for example, there's a housing co-operative especially set up for women over 50. They are 26 women between 50 and 80 who live in separate housing, but agree to do things as a community and look out for one another if they need help for a short time, to help people maintain their independence. Although there are only a small number of such housing co-operatives in the UK, there are more than 20 in development, including three for older LGBT women.

Shared lives

I spoke to Alex Fox who runs Shared Lives Plus. Shared Lives Plus is an umbrella body for homeshare schemes – this is where older people who need low-level help or companionship are matched with carefully vetted younger people who need somewhere to live. When a match is found, they move in and help out – with keeping on top of the garden, for example, or shopping or cooking. Often students are interested and it's a way – perhaps for around a year – of both people getting something out of sharing a space. Under these schemes – there are around 20 homeshare organisations in the UK and the number's growing rapidly – an agreement between the two people is drawn up, and the homeshare organisation will check in from time to time to make sure things are working out. Both people pay a small fee each week, up to £30, but in some places it's more for the younger person and less for the older. It's not rent; of course people are free to do that privately in a commercial relationship, but homeshare is different, for mutual benefit. That includes the older person feeling that they are helping a young person get a good start in life – a way for people to feel useful! And it provides basic human companionship in a way that, for example, befriending schemes don't. It's a relationship of equals. Currently there are around 400 of these kinds of homeshare arrangements in the UK (it's a much bigger movement in other countries like France, Spain and Portugal). If you're interested in this for yourself or want to suggest it to older friends or relatives, look on the Homeshare UK website, which will point you to schemes in your area to contact.

Of course, this 'shared lives' idea happens without any organisations being involved and given the pressures of housing and rent costs, many parents are living with adult children in later life. Having care and companionship from family members could be an ideal scenario – though that rather depends on how easygoing both parties are. In Singapore, where a comprehensive strategy to make the country respond positively to an ageing population has been drawn up, a new law is being introduced: The Maintenance of Parents Act. The Act compels adult children to pay maintenance to look after their over-60s parents if they're unable to subsist on their own. I'm not sure how something similar would go down in the UK, but as noted in the section later on caring for others, many millions of people are already caring for parents in their later life, and do it happily, and with love (even if perhaps both parent and 'child' occasionally have to bite their tongues!).

****

Home is so special to all of us, whether it's a flat or a mansion. Most of the time we take it for granted, pushing the hoover round every week or so and occasionally splashing out on some new cushions or saving up for a new sofa. Some people are big renovators, not batting an eyelid at taking on a 'Grand Designs' scale project. Most of us are happy with the odd lick of paint every couple of years to brighten things up.

But very little thought, discussion or publicity is given to how we will need to live as we age; how our house needs to work for us so we can stay mobile and use it all well, and how we'll manage our space. There's lots in the news about care homes – but what about other ways of living? This could include sharing your later life with people who could do some of the tasks that might have become difficult for you. It could mean moving to a retirement village or sharing your life with family, friends or young people who could benefit from low or no rent. As a minimum, if you stay in your own home it's certainly worth thinking about 'future-proofing' your home with adaptations, particularly if you move to a new house in middle age.

9

FRIENDS, FAMILY AND OTHER FOLK

So far we've looked at finances, your home and neighbourhood, your health, and what you'll do with your extra hours, days and years. But we haven't addressed something absolutely vital: your relationships. For most of us, whatever age or stage of life we're at, the state of our relationships is what will make the difference between feeling contented and feeling less happy with our lot. Feeling loved, connected to others, and having people to rely on is a fundamental human need, and when it's out of balance it affects all the other aspects of life – work and leisure, finances and health. Ultimately, we are social animals and the stuff of life is our personal relationships.

Replenishing the convoy

So, what are the implications for our relationships with others as we grow older? While friends, family and having a 'significant other' are important at any age, having people you rely on will become more important as the years go by, so we need to have an eye on the future, not just on life now.

I talked to Chris Sherwood, the Chief Executive of Relate, a charity that provides support and advice for people when relationships become difficult. He had some great advice about how to maintain relationships, thoughts on being single, how to think about a 'relationship MOT', preparing for retirement and therefore potentially spending more time with your partner, what to do about divorce, and some key things to remember.

> 'The first thing I'd say about relationships and later life is that it's not about the number of friends you have – it's about quality not quantity. Women are more likely to have fewer friends but have deeper connections with them, and the opposite is true for men. The main action we need to take is to "replenish the convoy" – by which I mean the people who are on the journey with you through life. The convoy could and should be made up of people of different ages, who mean different things to you, and could range from neighbours you speak to frequently to your life partner. Nurture all of those relationships and build new ones – people will fall away from the convoy, and others will join it. Some older people do feel lonelier when friends die – but you can make and nurture new friendships through volunteering, church groups, political party activity, and online networks.'

If you're single, should you be looking for a partner?

> 'Only if you want to! But remember, creating, forming and sustaining relationships is a skill – this goes for new friendships as well as new romantic relationships. We often think that finding and keeping friends or partners is just something we're good at or not – it's in our bones – but in fact it's a life skill that can be learnt. And the best way of learning how to connect better with people, to support friends and your partner, is by being in relationships and being reflective of how you behave with others. If you're single, and you want to get together with someone, go for it! Internet dating is very popular now and while it can be disheartening sometimes it can also be great fun.'

What should couples be wary of at retirement stage?

'A common issue that we're presented with at Relate is that people think a lot about saving and planning for retirement and have forgotten entirely to think about their relationship. Suddenly they're spending all their time with someone they hardly know any more. It's a good idea before you get to that stage to do a kind of MOT on your relationship – kick the tyres a bit. Talk about it – maybe go for a date night?'

Chris suggests that these are the things you could cover in a Relationship MOT:

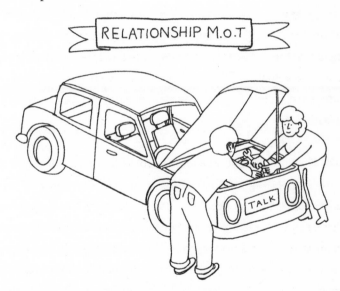

- Find **things you can do together** that you both like, so you're spending time doing something fulfilling. My partner and I love gardening, it's a really nice thing to do together.
- Equally important is **each of you having outside interests** independent of each other – so you have lots of stories to tell each other (and you're not spending absolutely all your time together!).

- Talk about **how satisfied you feel with the relationship**. This might be a hard one – remember to be sensitive and diplomatic. If there's something bothering you, don't let it boil away under the surface.
- **Sex is important**. Most people want to continue having sex as they grow older! Even if the urgency goes, the quality of your sex life will still be important – find ways to spice it up.
- **Commit to communicating well** in non-defensive and positive ways. You're both there for love and support – give as well as take.

Divorce rates are declining among most age groups, but rising in mid and later life, with the number of women over 60 divorcing rising by 38 per cent between 2005 and 2015 and a 23 per cent rise in men over 60 divorcing. Make of that what you will. It's worth noting as well that these statistics apply only to opposite-sex marriages and do not include information about dissolution of civil partnerships or same-sex marriages.

I asked Chris what happens when things go wrong with relationships.

'Indeed, there's the so-called silver splitter phenomenon, with divorce rates rising in people's 50s. With this, the important thing is to get support early. People wait up to six years in my experience to get help – if there are issues beyond the normal ups and downs of a relationship, talk to someone or use our Relate self-help tools. If you are getting divorced, prepare well. Think about assets you may need to unwind; there may be children and pets to think about, joint savings, pensions or house assets – talk to a lawyer and family mediator early on. And don't forget to get therapeutic help as separation processes are often painful. And do what's right for you afterwards – you don't need to jump into another relationship – you might want to focus on your friendships for a while, for example.'

I asked Chris to leave us with some key things to remember.

'One of the things I love about our society is that there's increasing choice about how to organise our relationships. You could have a husband, wife, civil partner, boyfriend or girlfriend or be happily single. You could be in a traditional or blended family, have children, or have great relationships with nieces, nephews and goddaughters/ sons. You could have lots of diversity in your convoy or be happy with a few close friends. It all comes back to quality – people in poor-quality relationships that are abusive are some of the worst-off people in society – and even on a broader community level, if you have a good quality of interaction with your neighbours (as opposed to say living next to people for 20 years and never talking to them), then those connections will simply help you and them be happier. So, I'll leave you with three things to remember about relationships, that are critical to preparing to have a good later life:

1. Nurture your convoy
2. Have a relationship MOT
3. Invest in your sex life!'

The Relate website has a fantastic range of self-help tools, stories and live chat on their website with trained relationship councillors. If you think you need some help now or want advice in planning for the future in your relationships, do talk to them.

Only the lonely

The opposite of having a range of good-quality relationships is in the spotlight at the moment, and rightly so. *Loneliness is more dangerous for your health than smoking!* is the depressing headline of research that's found its way into public consciousness in the last couple of years. We are facing an 'epidemic of loneliness'. So much so that the

Government created a Minister for Loneliness in 2017. Charities run campaigns, particularly at Christmas time, showing heartbreaking photos and adverts of people sitting alone at home with only the TV for company, to help fundraise for older people. And it's true, loneliness is a problem in later life. The charity The Silver Line runs a phone line, which has had nearly 2 million calls since it started in 2015 and call volumes often peak in the late evening with people calling just to be able to say 'good night' to someone. Loneliness and depression can often go hand in hand. Is a life worth living if it's lived alone?

But there are sides to this story that just aren't told. It would appear that it's only or even mainly older people that are lonely, and that this is a phenomenon that's got much worse over time. In fact, younger people are just as likely to feel lonely – see this chart from the Community Life Survey 2017/18, published by the Department for Digital, Culture, Media and Sport.

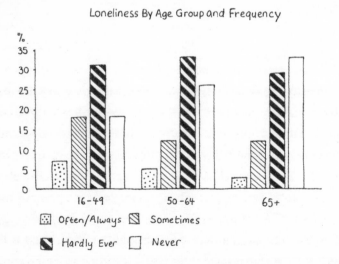

Loneliness By Age Group and Frequency

It shows that, in fact, the 16–49-year-old group experience loneliness more than over 65s. While this is a large age range, we know that people at the younger end (16–24) report more loneliness on average than much older age groups. If you look across life stages, you can see that there aren't huge differences in how lonely people feel.

This has remained relatively static over the years. It is perhaps because there is a larger number of older people in the population (including more 'much older' people, as we saw in Chapter One) that loneliness in people in later life seems more prominent now.

The other point about loneliness is that, for almost all of us, at points in our life we'll experience it. I know I have. It's just part of the human condition. And we also know, of course, that loneliness isn't just about the absence of other people; you can feel lonely in a group, or even in a close relationship.

So perhaps the story overall isn't so simple, and not so bad in terms of how you'll feel as you age.

I talked to Laura Alcock-Ferguson, Chief Executive of the Campaign to End Loneliness. Her perspective on loneliness was really insightful.

'Loneliness is a part of life. At different times in our existence we've had loneliness triggered for different reasons. In the past this could have been warring factions leaving people isolated. Now there's a different kind of fragmentation in society. People often live away from friends and other family members and there's less opportunity for them to be connected. The number of times we're actually with people has been massively impacted by social media and smartphone technology – a "like" on Facebook is not the same as a bear hug from someone you love. If you're alone, and feeling lonely, acknowledge it but go easy on yourself. As John Cacioppo said, loneliness is like hunger – a signal that you need to talk to someone, to connect – like hunger prompts you to eat.

'So there's social loneliness, missing being part of a crowd, which you can change by getting involved with activities locally; and there's emotional loneliness – missing intimacy and one or two close people. There's a whole spectrum of responses to feeling loneliness of any kind. You can ignore it and live with it. You can ask for support and take action, from joining a local club to seeking counselling. Exercise and a routine where you do things for yourself can help. Any option, and certainly any big change, needs lots of energy and commitment, and sometimes huge amounts of bravery and resilience. So, take it easy on yourself, acknowledge how you're feeling, and if you want to feel less lonely, know that you can make that change.'

Here are questions to mull over: For you personally, or for older friends or relatives, can loneliness be prevented? If you do feel lonely, can you 'treat' it? What can be done?

- Be aware of how you're feeling – take time to reflect and consider whether you feel happy/sad most of the time, whether you feel connected to others, and whether the things you do give you satisfaction, or make you feel anxious or isolated.
- Talk about it. Talking about loneliness has been really stigmatised, despite most of us feeling it at some point in our lives. Talk about it to friends, family members, health professionals. At the very least they will listen, and also may be able to empathise and share their own experiences of loneliness and ways they have coped with it.
- Be with others – there are many ways to do this, from joining a club/ evening class/exercise group, to specific "befriending" schemes. Volunteering is a great way to spend time with others and contribute to your community.
- Take it easy on yourself. Don't put yourself under pressure to make lots of new friends, go on hundreds of online dates, or volunteer for everything. Periods of loneliness will often pass; find things to do that will make you happy in yourself, even if they are things you do just by yourself!

Pets rock

British people love their pets (according to one survey – admittedly done by a pet insurance company!). Eighty-eight per cent of us say that we treat our pets the same as our children, and 60 per cent of pet owners said that they buy treats every week for their animal. And there's some evidence that having a pet can reduce loneliness. Having a dog can obviously encourage people to get out of the house every day, and possibly make it easier to talk to other people. Recently, the pet food company Pedigree joined forces with the Campaign to End Loneliness to help match older people who say they're lonely with dogs in their local area to combat isolation.

For physical activity, for companionship, could a dog, cat, rabbit or a herd of alpacas be fun in later life?

Being a carer

Loneliness is becoming well recognised as something we need to tackle, but there's a major area of life for millions of people in the UK that has had much less press: being a carer. Many people wouldn't say they are a 'carer' – they'd say they're looking after someone or helping out. It's not something that people plan for – but most people will do it at some time in their lives. It could mean looking after someone with a health condition – a partner, parents, or a sibling. Most people just aren't prepared for this, and while it can be rewarding, it can also be emotionally and practically challenging. But there are many things you can do to keep mentally and physically healthy, as well as manage finances and your time while caring for someone.

Carers UK's Emily Holzhausen passed on some tips:

'Go to the Carers UK website and use the Upfront Guide to Caring tool – it takes about 10 minutes and you come out with a tailored caring plan. And get a financial health check that includes what benefits you might be entitled to as a carer; again, the Carers UK website can help.

'If you're juggling work and care, talk to your employer about flexibility. If you've worked there six months or more you have the right to ask about flexible working – check the policies they have in place for time off for care in an emergency (they might be under special leave, or unpaid leave).

'For many people, caring can have an impact on your mental health. The stress of responsibility plus organising care, making appointments and so on (as well as living the rest of your life) can be tough, and some caring (for example, looking after someone with a mental health condition) can be stressful by its nature. Thinking about your own physical health, caring can be exhausting, and it's hard to find time for yourself to go to an exercise class, for example. The key thing is to look after yourself – get support that will give you some time for yourself. This could take many forms – formal support from a carer coming in, a day centre, or technology that helps you communicate with the person you're caring for if you can't be there in person, for example. If you can afford it, it's possible to buy in care support – use an accredited agency.'

Think about power of attorney, wills and other legal issues in advance – there's more about this area later in this chapter. If you're one of the 6.5 million carers in Britain at the moment, remember to take care of yourself too.

****

Relationships come in all shapes and sizes – from deep lifelong friendships to the once a year Christmas card list pal; from your second cousin twice removed to your 'significant other'. All are important in one way or another.

In a nutshell – whether you're an introvert or an extrovert, or like most of us, somewhere in between, we depend on other people. We need someone to turn to when times are hard, and someone to laugh at that extremely funny joke we've just thought up. Even though many people will have periods of loneliness in their life, this doesn't need to be a permanent state of affairs. Sharing your life and insights and connecting with people is something fundamental in human nature. Nurturing your close relationships and meeting other people socially – 'replenishing the convoy' – is really important. So as much as planning financially, and planning for your home and health, plan to have the kind of people around you that you want and relationships that suit you in later life.

Death and bereavement

Death. It's the only inevitable thing about life. It will happen to every single one of us. And yet most people barely think about it, and certainly don't want to talk about it with family or friends. Perhaps it's because research by a Christian think tank found that nearly half of people in Britain believe there is another life after death. Does this mean the other half are also at ease with the mystery, with the strange knowledge that one day we'll exist, and the next day we will not? Does the idea scare you – or are you already at peace with what will happen? Do you have a clue about the practical side of dealing with the death of a loved one, or how you might deal with your emotions about someone else's passing, or indeed your own, when you reach your final months, weeks and days? This section will help, both on the emotional and practical fronts.

But first, some views on death from different sources. A colleague at the Centre for Ageing Better asked her forthright four-year-old cousin, Kayleigh, some questions about death. She had some trenchant answers:

Kayleigh, what happens when you die?
'You can't move any more. If you die, you can't walk any more.'

Why can't you walk any more?
'Because you don't have a body, it's in the park. You put it in a box and put loads of mud on it, and worms eat your face.'

In the park?
'Yes, in the dead people's park.'

Oh, a cemetery?
'Yeah, a cemetery. You can buy flowers and go and visit them, but they can't come out. When you're dead, you live in the dead people's park and you can't get out and you never see them ever again.'

So, how do you know someone's going to die?
'Their face is all wrinkly, and their hair goes white.'

A slightly different view of what happens after death was explained to me by a lovely woman who is a Church of England priest in North London.

'When talking to a member of the congregation or anyone with a Christian faith, who's either facing death themselves or thinking about the death of a loved one, I ask them what their personal theology of death is – what they think happens. And I explain mine. I believe there is an afterlife that is a good place, where we can be reunited with people who have gone before us. Jesus is there, as is written in the scriptures.

'It really varies in terms of what people believe – and we talk about death a lot in the Church. When talking with family particularly about the kind of service that's right for them to grieve and celebrate the life of their loved one, there are different prayers to choose from in the funeral service. Even if you are not a Christian, you can ask for a funeral service in your parish CofE church – there must be prayers and a Bible reading, but we can tailor the service. These can be really different – I have had West Indian funerals, for example, where someone's played Amazing Grace on the saxophone and there were hymns sung at the graveside.

'Funerals are a celebration of life in many ways, and death an important part of the Christian faith – we celebrate God who was among us, incarnated as a man who both grieved for his friends and died himself. Whatever people's personal beliefs, I think we should talk about death more, and church is a good place to do it!'

If you want to say goodbye to a loved one without any mention of religion, a humanist funeral ceremony might be something to consider. Julia Whittaker has carried out funerals as a humanist celebrant and talked to me about what it involves.

'Humanists will give comfort and the ability for family and other loved ones to celebrate someone's life without God. We'll talk about and share memories of the person who's passed away, concentrating on what was good and what people loved about them, valuing what they did when they were alive. Sometimes families will read poems, and often there's some music special to the group. We'll have some quiet time to reflect on the life of the person who's passed away, then formally say goodbye to them.

'People have the choice about how to celebrate the life of their special friend. I went to one humanist funeral where the advance wishes of the person who'd died was that everyone should have champagne at the graveside after the coffin was lowered! Nature often plays a role. When my own daughter died, we planted an apple tree to remember her. There are so many ways to celebrate the life of someone who has died and remember them with love, without any reference to religion.'

Spiritual healing

As so often in life, bottling up our feelings and taking the 'stiff upper lip' approach doesn't work that well, and that's most true when we're coping with a loved one dying, or news that we don't have much longer to live. Talking about death, thinking about it, making plans and seeking support all help.

Felicity Warner is part of a growing movement of Soul Midwives, a community of around 800 people who are trained in helping people who are dying, and their families, particularly with the emotional and spiritual side of this final transition. Many work in hospices and hospitals. Some charge a fee, some volunteer. The trend is for soul midwives to become independent practitioners in communities, helping people plan for their final weeks and days and supporting people at the end of life. An increasing number of medical staff are training as soul midwives to complement their clinical skills. Felicity explained how people normally experience the news that they will soon die and what she and others can do to support them, with great advice for families and carers too.

'Death comes in so many guises, and while we expect a soft unravelling of life, even in old age death can come out of the blue. It can be easier for people if death is preceded by a gradual decline rather than something dramatic, but particularly if dementia is involved, the loss of the sense of who you are as well as the loss of function can be more difficult. We see, and help people, as they go through three distinct stages when they understand they are going to die, usually after a diagnosis of a terminal condition.

'The first stage we recognise is **chaos**. Someone is told they only have so long left to live and this usually prompts a period of chaotic distress. Plans are up in the air, people are sometimes in shock, and don't know what to do. There's too much to think about; it's literally a life-changing moment, and the rug has been pulled from under their feet. This phase can last anything from a few weeks to five or six months, and many also keep trying to have as normal a life as possible – socialising, having treatment and so on. We will help people by "holding the space" – being calm and steady, being there for people while they go through the distress. Then we'll start building them up, giving them comfort and advice and starting to help them put together a plan for how they will spend their remaining time. This is totally personal to them. A lot of people think they should do what they're told – that they will have to die in a hospice or hospital, for example, even if they would like to die at home. Have input where you can into these decisions – it's your death! It may be possible with the right infrastructure and support to die at home, for example, if that's what you want. Who do you want with you and who would you rather not see as you prepare for the end? The plan may also include practical items on resuscitation or antibiotics/tube feeding and your choice about whether or not you want these things. The plan should be workable, and flexible. Once out of the chaos stage, and the shock passes, people will sometimes change their minds about what they want, when they've had time to think it through more and feel more empowered about taking charge of their own way of dying.

'Then the person who's poorly goes into a second stage: **surrender**. It's a calmer time, physically and mentally. They accept that death will come, have more comfort about having a plan for it, and realise they can't stop the tide coming in. They start to go with the flow. We continue to support people in making their plans happen and helping them change them if they wish.

'Right at the end, in the last week or few days of life, people enter into a **transcendence** phase where, if all has gone well, their affairs are in order and they feel closure, they are ready to go. They hope to leave behind good memories for people who know them and will say, "It's time now. I am ready." They're at peace with their life and its ending. But some people never reach this stage. Some stay in "chaos" right until the end and cling on, which can be distressing for them and for their family. Indeed, many families think the right thing to do is rally round and try and keep their loved one alive at all costs. This is often very unhelpful. We need to understand how to manage our feelings and say it's okay to go now – it helps our loved one at their end and will help with our own grieving process.

'Of course, these stages can be different in length and intensity for everyone, and a lot depends on your medical condition and those around you, but we see this pattern of chaos, surrender and transcendence very often. It can be fulfilling and a very positive experience to help people through these stages.

'But most people aren't aware of what might happen and how they might feel. We simply need to prepare people more for death and grieving. We have a National Childbirth Trust in England for mothers and babies; why not an equivalent for the end of life?'

So, what should we do to prepare ourselves and our families for the inevitable?

- Go to one of the introduction days run by soul midwives or 'death doulas'; dip your toe in and have a discussion about where and how you might like to die. Take back your thoughts on a sheet of paper and stick it on the fridge with a magnet – make it a conversation point for the family; it doesn't have to be doom-laden, but it really is good to talk.
- Death cafés are a network of groups – meetings where people can talk about death – for people who are recently bereaved, are coping with someone who is dying, or who know they have a terminal condition. They are free, and at the time of writing, there are regular meetings of death cafés in Croydon, Kendal and Cambridge, with a pop-up café in Bristol. They also welcome people who are just curious and want to chat, learn, and understand more about the process of death and dying.

- As part of your emotional preparation, you might want to tie up loose ends, but the idea of resolving everything before you die might not be achievable, so on this as with other plans, it's important not to put yourself under too much pressure. You might want to tell people of your love, travel to a place that holds meaning, say farewell to family and friends, and perhaps forgive people their trespasses.

- If a loved one is dying, make sure you take care of yourself as well as thinking about them. Don't let yourself get burnt out in coping; looking after your own needs is not a weakness, it's essential.

- Age UK's pamphlet 'Let's talk about death and dying' has lots of good ways to start the conversation and advice on what to think about in the run-up to and after the death of an older friend or relative, and Independent Age has great leaflets and online advice as well.

I asked Felicity a final question, an existential one and maybe the reason why we fear talking about death. How can we live with the idea that one day – with no certainty about when – we are alive, and the next day we just stop existing? Her response was a gentle, but positive reminder to deeply value life:

'In their dying days, many people have expressed this to me differently. If we live our lives to the absolute full, life has a stronger feeling than death does. Most people do not regret their lives if lived well. You should enjoy life absolutely to the fullest, then when death comes, it will be palatable, it will be acceptable.'

Dying – the practical stuff

While emotional and spiritual preparation is fundamentally important, of course there are lots of elements to think about practically. Making sure you have made a will and perhaps have given your children or partner lasting power of attorney in the event you become too ill to make decisions will help with your emotional state as well – for you and your loved ones to have a calm and positive end. Here are the key areas to consider:

- You'll know this one – it's so important: make a will. If you haven't got one, do this now. Don't wait until you're much older or become ill. You can use a solicitor or there are do-it-yourself will-writing packs you can buy. A group of well-known charities run 'free wills month' every year where you can have a local solicitor help with your will for free (look online at freewillsmonth.co.uk). Remember to amend your will if you have a change in circumstances like getting married, entering into a civil partnership or buying a house with a partner.

- Make a note of all your bank accounts, insurance policies, pensions and important documents, and ensure that someone you trust has those details.

- Make clear who you want to make decisions for you if you're not able to do so. This might not be the person who the law recognises as your next of kin. Most hospitals and healthcare facilities will recognise who you nominate as the person who they should turn to if needed – though some may not. So, it's important, especially if you think there might be disagreements over who should make decisions on your behalf, that you make your wishes known to those around you, and in writing if possible. Although most places will ask you for your legal next of kin, i.e. spouse or nearest blood relative, they often simply mean 'who do I contact in an emergency?'. Feel free to ask what the question means in practice, and state who you view as closest to you. You can also order a card from Living Together, which you can carry with you, to make clear to NHS workers who you want to be considered your next of kin.

- If you're ill, talking to your family about how you want to die may not be enough in itself – for example, a Do Not Resuscitate order has to be written down in medical notes. And you should know that DNR only specifies that you don't want to be resuscitated if your heart stops, not that you don't want any invasive treatments, or that doctors won't do everything else they can to prolong your life. You might additionally consider making an Advance Decision, or Living Will, a decision you can make now to refuse specific types of treatment in the future. It lets family, carers and health professionals know what's acceptable to you. You might not want CPR, or ventilation, or antibiotics if you have a life-threatening infection, for example. If this is properly conveyed in legal documentation, doctors must respect this. You can create your own form, using the great website My Decisions, which is run by the charity Compassion in Dying. Forms can be completed online or downloaded and need to be signed and witnessed.

- Understand powers of attorney. Essentially, these are legal documents that allow you to appoint a representative to act for you in certain circumstances, usually under your control. However, a special type of power, a lasting power of attorney, allows your representative to make decisions for you if you become unable to do so and is frequently used by older people contemplating a future in which they may become physically or mentally incapable. A lasting power of attorney can be one or both of: power to make decisions about your **property and financial affairs** and/or power to make decisions on your **health and welfare**. The person making the power of attorney is called a donor, and the person appointed to act on their behalf is called an attorney. In order for you (or a parent, for example) to grant a power of attorney, you need to have the mental capacity to do so. You also need to think very carefully about who you trust enough to perform this important role. To grant a lasting power of attorney, you need to download and fill in one or both of the forms available on Gov.uk. You can do this yourself or get the help of a solicitor.
- Think about where you want to end your life. As noted above, hospice, home and hospital are all options, depending on your state of health.
- When someone dies, if the death was expected, and at home, call a doctor and a local funeral director, who normally have a 24-hour

service and will come out at any time. If the death was unexpected, it might need to be referred to the coroner – your GP will help with this. You'll need to get a medical certificate from the GP to register the death, which should be done within five days (eight days in Scotland).

Sue's story

Sue is in her 50s, and her parents lived long, healthy lives, but needed help when they reached their 80s. After it became apparent that her mother's memory was deteriorating, Sue's mum was referred to a memory clinic. But she didn't get a diagnosis of dementia – in some tests, she scored well, being able to count backwards from 100 in sevens, for example. At home, her cognitive decline was more apparent. She sometimes couldn't remember how to cook a chicken or who was coming over for dinner.

At the same time, Sue's father was also in ill health with a heart condition and found caring for his wife increasingly challenging. Her father's health worsened, and he died shortly after suffering a burst aneurysm. While believing that her father's pain could have been managed better, Sue thinks her father had a good death. His children could say goodbye and he was not in distress, saying he'd had a good life and was ready to go.

This left Sue and her family in charge of taking care of their mum. The family was uncertain whether Sue's mother's subsequent downturn was a response to her husband's death, or indicative of terminal decline. In the midst of this, Sue, a lawyer, knew that it could be helpful to have official documents relating to her mother's care, and her mother's GP advised that she was still able to understand the purpose of these. So, Sue and her siblings were granted lasting powers of attorney (LPA) over their mother's property and financial affairs as well as her health and welfare. The GP advised that a health and welfare LPA can be really important, for example with care facilities, which can sometimes be reluctant to share information about patients, even with family. They may be very careful about who they speak to, as not everyone in your family might agree on a course of action, so an LPA can make things a lot simpler.

How care homes work was a bit of a revelation for Sue, who had not expected there to be such a variety, and so little advice around. Because her mother was confused, residential homes were not keen to take her, but as she did not have an official diagnosis, dementia units were also not able to help or were inappropriate for her. Sue was able to find a home that provided initial residential care for her mum and also had a specialist dementia unit, which her mum moved to as her dementia progressed. Finally, as her condition deteriorated, and her physical needs moved beyond the capacity of the dementia unit, Sue had to move her mum to a nursing home. Having the LPAs at least made the decision-making process easier and gave Sue the power to decide where her mother could be best looked after and how to finance this. Sue's mum died some months later.

Sue's main recommendation for people in her position is to think about planning and to discuss your plans with your family. If you're updating your will, think about granting an LPA and who you'd like to appoint. A living will is also a good idea. If you don't have any children, it's particularly important to plan for a time when you might not be able to make your own decisions.

The final journey

As anthropologists will tell you, funeral rituals and our final resting places are one of the great distinguishing features of different cultures over time – from the great pyramid-topped tombs of the pharaohs to the New Orleans jazz funerals, we all have different ways to celebrate the passing of people we treasure. Here's what to think about when planning a funeral:

- A death has to be registered before a funeral can happen. If you want to bury or cremate the person quickly for cultural or religious reasons, funeral directors can arrange things very speedily.
- Family members sometimes have different views about how the funeral should be arranged – for example, the level of religious content. The vicar, priest or other religious officiator – or the humanist celebrant – can help

here, listening to the different wishes of relatives and helping people reach an agreement that makes everyone feel they can remember their loved one in a way that's important to them. The person themselves may have drawn up a letter of wishes, stipulating exactly what they want their funeral to be like (among other areas). This should sit alongside the will – but unlike the will isn't legally binding. Which? has a good guide to both wills and letters of wishes on its website.

- The average cost of a funeral is now around £4000 – bereavement is an expensive business. Your loved one may have had life insurance, savings set aside, or a prepaid funeral plan to cover this. If you're thinking about a prepaid plan, it's obvious advice to look closely at the terms and what the plan will actually buy – does it include a headstone, for example, if that's what you want or expect? And there are some dodgy ones out there, so if you want one, get one from a firm registered with the industry body that regulates funeral plan providers, the Funeral Planning Authority (no – I didn't know they existed either).

Funeral music charts

Co-op Funeralcare have been compiling 'the charts' of people's favourite funeral music, based on over 30,000 funerals in the UK.

- Over 40 per cent of people said they wanted music to make people laugh – which accounts for Monty Python's *Always Look on the Bright Side of Life* reaching the top 10.

- Adele's *Hello (From the Other Side)* is at number seven.

- People said they would consider having Queen's *Another One Bites the Dust*; *Going Underground* by The Jam; *Highway to Hell* (ACDC), and the Bee Gees' *Stayin' Alive*.

- Number one in the charts is consistently – you guessed it: *(I Did It) My Way*, by Frank Sinatra.

In some parts of the UK, you can use Tell Us Once – a service that informs most government organisations about someone's death, including HMRC, the DVLA, the DWP, the Passport office and the local authority. The registrar will give you the number for Tell Us Once when you register a death. This service doesn't operate in some places, for example, Brighton, Manchester or Northern Ireland, so there might be more calls to make if you don't live in an area covered by Tell Us Once. You'll need to tell the person's bank, utility companies, pension providers and any companies where they had subscriptions or memberships. When my own mum passed away I found that this was relatively easy, with banks and utility providers efficient and sympathetic.

If the person was living in their own home, you should contact their or your solicitor, who will help ensure the will is executed properly, and that, if they owned property, it would be included in the assets to be bequeathed. If they lived in private or socially rented accommodation, tell the landlord as soon as possible. If they lived in council housing, you must have removed their possessions and handed the keys back within a few weeks of their passing.

****

So – most of us know that death can be a sad and distressing experience, but much depends on the circumstances of the final few years, months and weeks. You can't prepare for a sudden death, but as it's one thing we're all sure about, there's lots you can do to prepare for your own end of life, and that of your loved ones, both practically, especially thinking about powers of attorney, and emotionally – beginning by talking about it! When the death of a loved one hits you hard, there are some very good support and counselling services out there, including Cruse Bereavement Care if you need them. And while we may deeply miss friends and family who have passed away, it's a reminder of our own mortality, and a gentle push for us to make the most of our own later lives...

10

MAKE CHANGE NOW

This book has ranged across the whole spectrum of planning for later life, from your own attitude to ageing, to financial security, how you will fill your days, your health, home, community and relationships. I hope it was an informative, interesting and sometimes fun read. So now you have a choice. To put it on a shelf, think, 'I'll do something about all that stuff in a few years' time', and get on with life at hand. Or to say to yourself, 'There are one or two things from this that I could probably get on with now, and I've been meaning to get around to, like writing my will, or putting a bit more into my pension.' Obviously, there's so much benefit in starting to take action in middle age for later life. Start small and grow those actions – into doing more for your health, perhaps to be more reflective about your attitude to getting older; into thinking about the design of your home and where you want to live; and into focusing on relationships and the wider community of people around you.

You might ask how much of all this advice do I follow myself? Good question! I am no superwoman, and I'm conscious that doing all of this, all at once, for anyone, would take superpowers in organisation, willpower and time management! But I will try and keep taking steps to change, and that's a good way for anyone to start. Writing this book, interviewing experts and 'ordinary people' alike has been a real journey of discovery for me. At times a fascinating journey, learning much more about the practical challenges – and brilliant opportunities – of my middle age and later life – and how to prepare for them. At times it's been an emotional one, particularly when talking to 'soul midwife' Felicity Warner; remembering the death of loved ones and being reminded that life is not for ever, so we must make the absolute best of it.

So, for me, and you, here's a brief checklist of things to think about, and make small – or big – changes in, to help make your later life great.

Your lifespan

Of course, no-one knows how long they're going to live. But you might be set for many more years than you think. If you're in middle age, realise that you could have 30 or more years ahead – and you'll probably live longer than your parents did. A good 'longevity' calculator might give you a more accurate idea of the possible length of your later life.

Your attitude towards getting older

Awareness about your own attitude to your ageing is key. Does growing older fill you with horror or do you welcome it with open arms? Being positive and accepting of ageing could be great for your health and even lead to longer life.

Your finances

It's head out of sand time. Work out how much income you want each year of your later life, and perhaps try to take into account some unforeseen circumstances like care costs. What does this mean for your financial behaviour now? How much have you got in your pension pots and other savings? Do you own your own house or have other assets? Perhaps working for longer and saving more is part of the answer to building up more pension and income if you want to be able to be financially comfortable in older age.

Your work and retirement plans

Working for longer – to state pension age and beyond – will help with financial security but has benefits in its own right. It gives many people meaning and purpose and can mean a sociable life full of stimulation and challenges. But if work's not good or fulfilling now, set out to change it if you can – try for more flexibility, retraining, working in a different field or even becoming self-employed. When it's time to think about retirement, prepare for it – emotionally as well as practically; what will you do? Volunteering and helping out in the community is a choice for many. And how will you manage changes in your relationships?

Your health

I have been going on and on about having a healthier diet, exercising more, stopping smoking and reducing alcohol. This is not to denigrate the pleasures of a great meal and a glass of wine, nor to perhaps oversell the endorphins you get from a 5km run. Small changes, including doing more strength and balance exercises, make a difference at any age. If you have one or more long-term health conditions, or deterioration of eyesight and hearing for example, get help to manage them well and of course your later life can still be a great time.

Your neighbourhood

People often take for granted the idea either that they'll stay put or that they'll make a big change – moving to the country or retiring to

Spain, for example. But any choice about which country, region, city, village or neighbourhood you choose to spend your later years in should be a conscious one. Will you feel part of a safe, positive community that has great services, transport links and is well designed? If you're not sure, check it out – and join in the Age-friendly Cities and Communities movement.

Your home

We value our homes so much, particularly if we're lucky enough to own one. But will we need to adapt it for later life? Simple and small changes could 'future-proof' your house and make it a lot easier to use. And there will be a range of options at the point you decide you want to move – from co-housing to a 'shared lives' arrangement, to a retirement village.

Your relationships

Underlying most people's happiness is having loving relationships and close friendships (and of course the opposite of this is dealing with loneliness if you or someone you know experiences it). Be conscious about 'replenishing your convoy' of people who travel life's journey with you – including perhaps being close to people of different ages. But don't stay with people who make you feel unhappy – and there's lots of support out there to help you through difficult times.

Your final preparation – and thinking about the death of loved ones

Death is part of life – the inevitable part that people don't really talk about. It's worth thinking more about the practical elements of preparation for when your parents, partner or other loved ones die, including wills (for you as well!), and powers of attorney, as well as understanding advance directives in case the need arises. And remember that letting go will be a final act of love; and that there's help to work through grief if you need it.

I hope that final chapter will be many years away for you – so let's get planning to make the best of those years. Good luck and have a great later life!

TOP RESOURCES

General Resources

Gov.uk, www.gov.uk
Citizens Advice, www.citizensadvice.org.uk

One: The 'new' issue of old age

BBC and Aviva Life Expectancy calculators, *to find out how many years you've got left to enjoy*, www.bbc.co.uk/news/health-44107940, www.ons.gov.uk/peoplepopulationandcommunity/healthandsocialcare/healthandlifeexpectancies/articles/whatismylifeexpectancyandhow mightitchange/2017-12-01

Two: How are you ageing?

Centre for Ageing Better, *publications on what needs to change in society to prepare for ageing*, www.ageing-better.org.uk/publications

Three: Are you an old age ageist?

Positive Ageing, *tips on how to embrace ageing in a positive way*, positiveageing.org.uk
Age UK, *for more information on ageism, and your legal rights, as well as a host of other resources*, www.ageuk.org.uk
Robert Butler, *Why Survive? Being Old in America*, Harper and Row: New York, 1975. Butler's book provides a snapshot of ageing in the US in the 1970s, and what institutions and Americans themselves need to do to make longer lives fulfilling ones.

Robert Butler and M.I. Lewis, *Love and Sex After 60*, Ballantine:
New York, 1993. A guide to intimacy and relationships in later life.

Four: Funding it

Pensions Advisory Service, *get independent advice about pension
savings*, www.pensionsadvisoryservice.org.uk

Pension Wise, *a government-run service, you can book appointments over
the phone or online to discuss your pension plans*, www.pensionwise.
gov.uk/en

Age UK, *for information on the risks and benefits of equity release*, www.
ageuk.org.uk/information-advice/money-legal/income-tax/equity-
release/

Citizens Advice, *advice on topics from benefits to pensions and everything
in between, you can also find your nearest CAB centre* www.
citizensadvice.org.uk

Independent Age, *provides advice on topics relevant to remaining
independent in older age, including money and benefits*, www.
independentage.org

Transport Scotland, *for information on concessionary travel for over 60s
and disabled people*, www.transport.gov.scot/concessionary-travel

NI Direct, *provides information on over 60 concessionary passes, and
all-Ireland travelcards for the over 65s*, www.nidirect.gov.uk/articles/
free-and-concessionary-bus-and-rail-travel

Five: Nice work if you can get it

WEA, *for finding learning opportunities in your local area*, www.wea.
org.uk

UnLtd, *fund and support social entrepreneurs*, www.unltd.org.uk

FutureLearn, *for online classes in a range of subjects*, www.future
learn.com

OpenLearn, *provides free online educational resources, including hundreds of free classes*, www.open.edu/openlearn

University of the Third Age, *to find classes run by, and attended by, retired and semi-retired people*, www.u3a.org.uk

Carers UK, *for help and advice on managing care for yourself and others*, www.carersuk.org

National Careers Service, *provides information and advice on learning, training and works, including a skills health check*, nationalcareersservice.direct.gov.uk

NVCO and **National DO IT**, *for volunteering opportunities*, www.ncvo. org.uk *and* do-it.org

GP at Hand, *an app-based GP practice, which operates mainly via video consultations*, www.gpathand.nhs.uk

AbilityNet, *provides information and advice on how to adapt and adjust technology for users with additional needs*, www.abilitynet.org.uk/ we-are-abilitynet-adapting-technology-changing-lives

Online Centres Network, *to find your local online centre and improve your digital skills*, www.onlinecentresnetwork.org

Six: Fit as a fiddle or good enough health?

Diabetes UK, *for advice on coping with diabetes and to find local support*, www.diabetes.org.uk

The NHS website, *a health information service with a Health A–Z, advice on living well and a guide to social care and support*, www.nhs.uk

British Heart Foundation, *information on how to prevent and cope with heart disease*, www.bhf.org.uk

Cancer Research UK, *look up how to reduce your risk, how to cope with a diagnosis, and find a list of resources to help*, www.cancer researchuk.org

Macmillan Cancer Support, *offers physical, financial and emotional support for cancer patients and their families*, www.macmillan.org.uk

The Stroke Association, *for advice on how to live well after a stroke,* www.stroke.org.uk

Versus Arthritis, *for the latest research, treatments and exercises to help,* www.versusarthritis.org

British Lung Foundation, *tips on how to manage breathlessness and more about COPD and other lung conditions,* www.blf.org.uk

Alzheimer's Society, *latest research and advice on dealing with Alzheimer's and other types of dementia,* www.alzheimers.org.uk

Dementia UK, *offers specialist support, guidance and practical solutions to families living with dementia,* www.dementiauk.org

Dementia Friends, *an initiative to change people's perceptions of dementia,* www.dementiafriends.org.uk

Action on Hearing Loss, *practical tips to help people with impaired hearing,* www.actiononhearingloss.org.uk

Parkrun, *organisers of hundreds of local 5km runs weekly, you can find out more at* www.parkrun.org.uk

Lingo Flamingo, *an organisation that runs language classes all over Scotland for older people, designed to enhance cognitive function,* www.lingoflamingo.co.uk

MindEd, *an e-learning tool that aims to give you and your family advice on mental health,* mindedforfamilies.org.uk/older-people

Royal National Institute of Blind People, *the UK's largest sight loss charity, providing extensive advice on eye health as well how to cope with sight loss,* www.rnib.org.uk/

Menopause Matters UK, *provides up-to-date information about the menopause, symptoms and treatment,* www.menopausematters.co.uk

Eatwell Guide, *NHS advice on food, diet and digestive health, including recipes and tips,* www.nhs.uk/live-well/eat-well/the-eatwell-guide

M. Gray and D. Moran, *Sod Sitting, Get Moving! Getting Active in Your 60s, 70s and Beyond*, Green Tree: London, 2017, a guide to getting the most out of exercise in later life.

Seven: Where you'll live

Age-friendly Cities and Communities, *a global network established to promote healthy and active ageing*, www.who.int/ageing/projects/age_friendly_cities_network/en

AA, *for tips on how to keep driving safely for as long as you want*, www.theaa.com

Royal Society for the Prevention of Accidents, *for training courses and advice on how to improve your driving*, www.rospa.com

Cycling UK, *tips on how to start, and for local groups*, www.cyclinguk.org

Walking for Health, *a network of health walks in England to help people lead a more active lifestyle, with the support of specially trained volunteers*, www.walkingforhealth.org.uk

Police UK, *for information on crime rates and prevention in your local area*, www.police.uk

Better Mobility, *sells mobility equipment, and provides advice and resources for using them, as well as how to fund them*, www.bettermobility.co.uk/index.php

Eight: What your home should look like

Gov.uk, *for legal information on private renting*, www.gov.uk/private-renting

Shelter, *for advice on housing, including knowing your rights in the private and social renting sector*, www.shelter.org.uk

Homeshare, *the UK network for Homeshare organisations*, homeshareuk.org

Campaign to End Loneliness, *a campaign to encourage social connection and raise awareness of loneliness*, www.campaigntoendloneliness.org

Nine: Friends, family and other folk

Relate, *for advice on how to deal with relationships*, www.relate.org.uk

The Silver Line, *a 24-hour confidential helpline for older people*, www.thesilverline.org.uk

Death Cafés, *local events where you can talk about death and dying*, deathcafe.com

Cruse Bereavement Care, *a confidential and free service for the bereaved. You can speak to them face to face, online or on the phone*, www.cruse.org.uk

My Decisions, *this website will ask you questions about what you want and your beliefs to help you create advance decisions or an advanced statement*, mydecisions.org.uk/

Living Together, *advice for unmarried couples, who are not recognised by law as next of kin*, www.advicenow.org.uk/living-together

Compassion in Dying, *an organisation formed to help people plan ahead, providing information for older people, as well as carers and professionals*, compassionindying.org.uk/

Which?, *has a section dedicated to later life care, covering everything from benefit entitlements to advance decisions and wills*, www.which.co.uk/later-life-care

Funeral Planning Authority, *protecting consumers' interests in the prepaid funeral plan industry*, funeralplanningauthority.co.uk

Tell Us Once, *a service that enables you to report a death to most government organisations in one go*, www.gov.uk/after-a-death/organisations-you-need-to-contact-and-tell-us-once

ACKNOWLEDGEMENTS

An enormous thanks to the following people for contributions, corrections, advice and stories (listed in chapter order):

Hannah Swift, University of Kent

Guy Robertson, Positive Ageing Associates

Michelle Cracknell, Pensions Advisory Service

Hannah Mills, Lorraine Charlton and colleagues from Citizens
    Advice

The Transitions in Later Life learning community and the
    Calouste Gulbenkian Foundation UK

Alyson Bowcott and Legal and General

Shaun Delaney, NCVO

Dr Thomas Bak, University of Edinburgh

Alison Cox, Cancer Research UK

Felicity Barr and Diabetes UK

Alison Tedstone, Public Health England

Kate Sheehan, the Occupational Therapy Service

Alex Fox, Shared Lives Plus

Alison Armstrong, Whiteley Village

Chris Sherwood, Relate

Laura Alcock-Ferguson, Campaign to End Loneliness

Emily Holzhausen, Carers UK

Julia Whittaker, humanist celebrant

Felicity Warner, Soul Midwife

Christopher Jenkins

Many individuals who agreed to talk to me or allow me to use their stories, including Nora Doleman, Bob Dunkerley, Pat Scully, Liz

Clutterbuck, Peggy Ruff, and many others who spoke anonymously, whose words I hope will inspire others.

All the staff at the Centre for Ageing Better, particularly Amy McSweeney, who provided invaluable research support, Jess Kuehne and Luke Price for fact-checking; and all the Trustees, particularly Mark Hesketh for his contribution on the finances chapter.

BIBLIOGRAPHY

Introduction

Cancer Research UK, How Smoking Causes Cancer, 2016.

Department for Work and Pensions, Workplace pension participation and saving trends: 2006 to 2016, Table 1.1: Eligible employees participating in workplace pensions by sector, Percentage of eligible employees participating 2006–2016.

Fujiwara, D., Oroyemi, P. and McKinnon, E., 'Wellbeing and Civil Society: Estimating the value of volunteering using subjective wellbeing data', Department for Work and Pensions, 2013.

Grimby, G. and Saltin, B., 'The ageing muscle', *Clinical Physiology*, 3(3), pp.209–218, 1983.

Jones, D., Young, A. and Reeder, N., 'The benefits of making a contribution to your community in later life', Evidence Briefing, Centre for Ageing Better, 2016.

Levy, R., Slade, M.D., Kunkel, S.R. and Kasl, S.V., 'Longevity Increased by Positive Self-Perceptions of Aging', *Journal of Personality and Social Psychology*, Vol. 83, No. 2, pp. 261–270, 2002.

Lloyd, J., 'Older Owners Research on the lives, aspirations and housing outcomes of older homeowners in the UK', London: Strategic Society Centre, 2015.

McNeill, A., Brose, L., Calder, R., Bauld, L. and Robson, D., Evidence review of e-cigarettes and heated tobacco products, A report commissioned by Public Health England', London: Public Health England, 2018.

NHS, Exercise for Older Adults, www.nhs.uk/live-well/exercise/physical-activity-guidelines-older-adults/, 2018.

NHS Digital, Statistics on Smoking in England – 2017, Table 3.5 – Total
   registered deaths, deaths from diseases that can be caused by smoking,
   and those estimated to be attributable to smoking, for adults aged 35
   and over, by gender, 2017.

NHS Digital, Health Survey for England, Trend tables – 2010–16.

Office for National Statistics, Pensioners' incomes series: financial year
   2016/17, Table 3.10: The percentage of pensioner units with private
   pension income and the average amount for those in receipt, 1994/95–
   2016/17.

Office for National Statistics, Statistics on Smoking, England – 2017,
   Table 1. Proportion of cigarette smokers, by sex and age, England,
   2000 to 2017.

Chapter One: The 'new' issue of old age

Adams, D., Swift, H., Lamont, R. and Drury, L. (2015), 'The barriers
   to and enablers of positive attitudes to ageing and older people,
   at the societal and individual level', Future of an ageing
   population: evidence review. Foresight: Government Office for
   Science.

BBC, 'How long are you going to live?', May 2018.

Christensen, K., Doblhammer, G., Rau, R. and Vaupel, J.W., 'Ageing
   Populations: The Challenge Ahead', The Lancet, Volume 374, No. 9696,
   pp. 1196–1208, 2009.

English Longitudinal Study of Ageing, Wave 8, 2018.

Fisher, H., Anatomy of Love: A Natural History of Mating, Marriage, and
   Why We Stray, New York: Random House, 1992.

Freeman, A., Tyrovolas, S., Koyanagi, A. et al, 'The role of socioeconomic status in depression: results from the COURAGE (aging
   survey in Europe), BMC Public Health, 16 (1098), 2016.

Office for National Statistics, Birth summary tables on England and
   Wales, 2017-based, Table 1, 2018.

Office for National Statistics, Changing trends in mortality: an international comparison: 2000 to 2016.

Office for National Statistics, Estimates of the population for the UK, England and Wales, Scotland and Northern Ireland, mid-2017, MYE1: Population estimates: Summary for the UK, mid-2017.

Office for National Statistics, Expectation of life, principal projection: 2016-based, England and Wales, figures based on 2018 cohort expectation of life, rounded to the nearest year.

Office for National Statistics, Health State Life Expectancies, 2015–2017: Life Expectancy at Birth and at Age 65, by Local Areas – UK, 2018.

Office for National Statistics, Average age at death – by sex, UK, 2018.

Office for National Statistics, National Population projections by single year of age, 2016-based.

Office for National Statistics, 'What is my life expectancy? And how might it change?', December 2017.

World Health Organization, Life expectancy and Healthy life expectancy data by WHO region, 2016.

Yip, J., Luben, R., Hayat, S., Khawaja, A., Broadway, D., Wareham, N., Khaw, K.T. and Foster, P.J., 'Area deprivation, individual socioeconomic status and low vision in the EPIC-Norfolk Eye Study,' *Journal of Epidemiological* and *Community Health* 68(3), 2014, pp. 204-2010.

Zaninotto. P Sacker. A and Head. J., 'Relationship Between Wealth and Age Trajectories of Walking Speed Among Older Adults: Evidence from the English Longitudinal Study of Ageing', *The Journals of Gerontology Series A Biological Sciences and Medical Sciences*, 68(12), 2013, pp. 1525–1531.

Chapter Two: How are you ageing?

Centre for Ageing Better/Ipsos MORI, Later life in 2015: An analysis of the views and experiences of people aged 50 and over, 2015.

Chapter Three: Are you an old age ageist?

Aspinall, A., 'Robot CATS to be used to help elderly people with tasks and reminders', *Daily Mirror*, 2017.

Baghot, M., 'Sex robots could be used by the elderly to help them overcome anxiety and erectile dysfunction', *Daily Mirror*, 2017.

Buchanan, K., (2013), 'Leading Men Age, But Their Love Interests Don't', Vulture.

Butler, R., 'Age-Ism: Another Form of Bigotry', *The Gerontologist*, 9(4), pp. 243–246, 1969.

Child, B., 'Maggie Gyllenhaal: At 37 I was "too old" for role opposite 55-year-old man', *Guardian*, 2015.

Commission on Older Women, Interim Report, The Labour Party, 2013.

Duffy, B., Shrimpton, H. and Clemence, M, 'Millennial Myths and Realities', London: Ipsos MORI, 2017.

English Longitudinal Study of Ageing, Wave 8, 2018.

Hughes, J., 'Forgetful elderly couple offer £100 reward if someone can find their car they lost FOUR days ago', *Daily Mirror*, 2018.

Keegan, S., 'Paranoid granny spends £4,000 defending her home against wi-fi signals', *Daily Mirror*, 2014.

Kelly, J., 'Pensioner "who doesn't like men" drives mobility scooter into one police officer and hits another with bottle', *Daily Mirror*, 2018.

Laidlaw, K., Kishita, N., Shenkin, S.D. and Power, M.J., 'Development of a Short-Form of the Attitudes to Ageing Questionnaire', *International Journal of Geriatric Psychiatry*, Vol. 33, pp. 113–121, 2018.

Levy, R., Slade, M.D., Kunkel, S.R. and Kasl, S.V., 'Longevity Increased by Positive Self-Perceptions of Aging', *Journal of Personality and Social Psychology*, Vol. 83, No. 2, pp. 261–270, 2002.

Shelmerdine, J. Jr., *Driven to Kill*, Channel 5, first broadcast 17 April 2014.

Unattributed, 'Pensioner dies after swallowing his wedding ring without knowing it', *Daily Mail*, 2010.

YouGov, 'Age Discrimination in the Workplace', commissioned by the Centre for Ageing Better, 2018.

Chapter Four: Funding it

Age UK, Carer's Allowance, 2019.

Age UK, 'Paying for Care and Support at Home', Factsheet 46, April 2018.

Bank of England, data from Statistical Interactive Database – official Bank Rate history, available at: www.bankofengland.co.uk/boeapps/iadb/Repo.asp, 2018.

BT, 'Odds of winning National Lottery Lotto jackpot lengthen with 59 balls', 2015.

Carers UK, Carer's Allowance Fact Sheet 2018/19, 2019 updates.

Carter, C., 'Pensioners travel length of Britain for free using bus passes', *Telegraph*, 2013.

Care Quality Commission, Cliffdale Rest Home Inspection report, 2016.

Care Quality Commission, The Fern Residential Home Inspection report, 2017.

Cavaglieri, C., Premium Bonds, *Which?*, 2018.

Citizens Advice, Benefits for Older People, 2018.

Citizens Advice, People in multiple jobs missing out on a workplace pension, reveals Citizens Advice, 2017.

Cliffdale Rest Home, Our Fees and Paying for Care, 2018.

Department for Work and Pensions Tabulation Tool, Great Britain: percentage of all claimants in receipt of the state pension, September 2014.

Department for Work and Pensions, Households below average income: An analysis of the UK income distribution: 1994/95 to 2015/16, Tables 6.1tr and 6.3tr, 2017.

Department for Work and Pensions, Income-related Benefits: estimates of take-up: financial year 2016/17, Tables PC1 and PC4, 2018.

Department for Work and Pensions, Stat Xplore, State pension caseload data, £ per week, November 2017.

Department for Work and Pensions, State Pension Age Review, July 2017 Report.

Department for Work and Pensions, Workplace pension participation and saving trends: 2006 to 2016, Table 1.1: Eligible employees participating in workplace pensions by sector, Percentage of eligible employees participating 2006–2016.

Duffy, B., 'On the money? Misperceptions and personal finance', Ipsos MORI, 2015.

Ferns Residential Home, Fees as of May 2018.

Gardiner, L., The Million Dollar Be-Question, Inheritances, gifts, and their implications for generational living standards, Resolution Foundation/Intergenerational Commission, 2017.

GOV.UK, Voluntary National Insurance, 2017.

Independent Age, Care Home Fees and Your Property, Fact Sheet, 2018.

Laing Buisson, Care of Older People, Market Report. 29th Edition: London, 2018.

Money Advice Service, Lifetime allowance for pension savings, 2018.

Money Advice Service, Why it pays to save regularly, 2017.

National Lottery, The Millionaire Map, 2018.

OECD, Pensions at a Glance: United Kingdom, OECD Publishing: Paris, 2017.

Office for National Statistics, Attitudes analysis by characteristics, July 2012 to June 2014, Great Britain, User Requested Data, Ref: 006201.

Office for National Statistics, Community Care Statistics: Social Services Activity, England 2013–14, Table 3.1.

Office for National Statistics, UK Population Estimates, 1838 to 2017, Table 6: Population estimates for Great Britain, by sex and single year of age, Mid-1961 to Mid-2017.

Page, B., 'What will make you happy? Concept, Measurement and Evidence', Ipsos MORI, 2018.

Pensions Advisory Service, The State Pension: What You Might Get, 2016.

Shropshire Council, Factsheet 7: Paying for your care and support, 2018, www.shropshire.gov.uk.

Wealthsmiths, S., The Generation Gap: Exploring the changing attitudes to inheritance and the implications for the financial services industry, 2017.

Chapter Five: Nice work if you can get it

AirBnB, Senior Hosts in Europe, Report read at: www.airbnbaction.com/wp-content/uploads/2016/09/Airbnb_SeniorHostsEuropeReport_English_9-13-16.pdf, 2016.

Azoulay, P., Jones, B., Kim, J.D. and Miranda, J., 'Age and High-Growth Entrepreneurship', MIT: Cambridge, Massachusetts, 2018.

Cabinet Office, Community Life Survey 2015/16: Statistical Press Release, 2016.

Centre for Ageing Better/Business in the Community, 'Becoming an Age-Friendly Employer', London: 2018.

Centre for Ageing Better and Calouste Gulbenkian Foundation, Evaluation of Transitions in Later Life Pilot Projects, summary and report available at: www.ageing-better.org.uk/publications/evaluation-transitions-later-life-pilot-projects-executive-summary, 2017.

Cridland, J., Independent Review of the State Pension Age: Smoothing the Transition, 2017.

Dawson, C., Henley, A. and Latreille, P., 'Why do individuals choose self-employment?', Institute for Study of Labor (IZA): Bonn, 2009.

Department for Business, Energy and Industrial Strategy, The Characteristics of those in the Gig Economy, figures from NatCen polling analysis, 2017.

Department of Health, Long Term Conditions, Compendium of Information: Third Edition. Figures based on 2010/11 Quality and Outcomes Framework and the 2009 General Lifestyle Survey, 2012.

Department for Digital, Culture, Media and Sport, Community Life Survey, 2017/18, Table D1: Formal Volunteering at least once a year and Table D2: Informal Volunteering at least once a year, 2018.

Department for Work and Pensions, Fuller Working Lives: A Partnership Approach, London: 2017.

Drydakis, N., MacDonald, P., Chiotis, V. and Somers, L., 'Age discrimination in the UK labour market. Does race moderate ageism? An experimental investigation', Applied Economics Letters 25(1), pp. 1–4.

Franklin, B., Beach, B., Bamford, S.M. and Creighton, H., 'The Missing Million: Illuminating the employment challenges of the over-50s'. London: BIT, 2014.

Jones, D., Young, A. and Reeder, N., 'The benefits of making a contribution to your community in later life', Evidence Briefing, Centre for Ageing Better, 2016.

Lloyds Bank, UK Consumer Digital Index: Benchmarking the Digital and Financial Capability of UK Consumers, 2016.

McKay, S. and Simpsons, I., Work: Attitudes and experiences of work in a changing labour market, British Social Attitudes, NatCen Social Research, Vol. 33, 2015.

OECD, Education at a Glance: Highlights, OECD Publishing: Paris, 2012.

Office for National Statistics, Job related training or education in the last 3 months, UK, April to March 2017. User requested data. Reference number: 007354. Using Annual Population Survey (April–March 2017) data.

Office for National Statistics, Labour Force Survey, A01: Summary of labour market statistics, Table 2: Labour market activity by age group (seasonally adjusted), August–October 2018.

Office for National Statistics, Leisure time in the UK: 2015, Figure 3: Mean leisure time per week by activity type and sex (whole population aged eight and over), UK, 2017.

Richardson, J., I Am Connected: New Approaches to Supporting People in Later Life Online, Good Things Foundation and the Centre for Ageing Better, 2018.

Yeun, W., Sidhu, S, Vassilev, G., Mubarak, S., Martin, T. and Wignall, J., Trends in Self-Employment in the UK, Office for National Statistics, 2018.

University of Cambridge, Retirement Policy, policy available at: www.hr.admin.cam.ac.uk/files/retirement_policy_2017.pdf, 2016.

University of Oxford, Employer Justified Retirement Age, policy available at: www.admin.ox.ac.uk/personnel/end/retirement/acrelretire8+/ejra/, 2017.

YouGov, Age Discrimination in the Workplace, commissioned by Centre for Ageing Better, 2018.

Chapter Six: Fit as a fiddle or good enough health?

Age UK, Incontinence, www.ageuk.org.uk/information-advice/health-wellbeing/conditions-illnesses/incontinence/, 2018.

Age UK, Your Mind Matters, 2016.

Ahmadi-Abhari, S., Guzman-Castillo, M., Bandosz, P. et al, Temporal trend in dementia incidence since 2002 and projections for prevalence in England and Wales to 2040: modelling study, *British Medical Journal: Clinical Research* 358 (2856), 2017.

Al-Qubaeissy, K.Y., Fatoye, F.A., Goodwin, P.C., Yohannes, A.M., The effectiveness of hydrotherapy in the management of rheumatoid arthritis: a systematic review, *Musculoskeletal Care*, 11 (1), pp. 2–18, 2013.

Alzheimer's Research UK, Types of dementia; Alzheimer's disease, 2016.

British Heart Foundation, CVD Statistics – BHF UK Factsheet, 2018.

Cancer Research UK, Statistics on Preventable Cancers, CRUK estimates available at: www.cancerresearchuk.org/health-professional/cancer-statistics/risk/preventable-cancers, 2016.

Claus, E., Schildkraut, J., Iversen, E.S., Berry, D. and Parmigiani, G., Effect of BRCA1 and BRCA2 on the Association Between Breast Cancer Risk and Family History, *Journal of the National Cancer Institute*, 90 (23), pp. 1824–1829, 1998.

College of Podiatry, Ageing Feet, www.scpod.org/foot-health/common-foot-problems/ageing-feet/, 2018.

Collins, R., Reith, C. and Emberson, J. et al, 'Interpretation of the evidence for the efficacy and safety of statin therapy', *The Lancet*, 388:10059, pp: 2532–2561, 2016.

Department of Health, Action Plan on Hearing Loss. London: NHS England, 2015.

Department of Health, How to keep health risks from drinking alcohol to a low level: Government response to the public consultation. London: Williams Lea, 2016.

Department of Health, The Musculoskeletal Services Framework: – A joint responsibility: doing it differently, 2006.

Department of Health, National Service Framework for Diabetes: Standards, 2001.

Dhalwani, N., O'Donovan, G., Zaccardi, F., Hamer, M., Yates, T., Davies, M. and Khunti, K., 'Long Term Trends of Multimorbidity and association with physical activity in older English population', *International Journal of Behavioural Nutrition and Physical Activity*, 13:8, 2016.

European Bone and Joint Health Strategies Project, European action towards better musculoskeletal health: A Public Health Strategy to Reduce the Burden of Musculoskeletal Conditions. The Bone and Joint Decade, Sweden, 2006.

Gatineau, M., Hancock, C., Holman, N. et al, *Adult Obesity and Type 2 Diabetes*. Oxford: Public Health England, 2014.

Godfrey, M., Literature and policy review on prevention and services. *UK Inquiry into Mental Health and Well-Being in Later Life*. London: Age Concern and Mental Health Foundation, 2005.

Grimby, G. and Saltin, B. 'The ageing muscle', *Clinical Physiology*, 3(3), pp.209–218, 1983.

Katz, D., Brown, J. and West, R., 'Real-world' effectiveness of smoking cessation treatments: a population study', *Addiction*, 109 (3), pp. 491–499, 2014.

Marcinkiewicz, A. and Reid, S., British Social Attitudes Survey: Attitudes to Dementia, Findings from the 2015 British Social Attitudes survey, Public Health England, 2015.

Meehan, M. and Penckofer, S., 'The Role of Vitamin D in the Aging Adult', *Journal of Aging and Gerontology*, 2 (2), pp. 60–71, 2014.

Lean, M.E., Leslie, W.S. and Barnes, A.C. et al, 'Primary care-led weight management for remission of Type 2 diabetes (DiRECT): an open-label, cluster-randomised trial', *The Lancet*, 391(10120), pp.541–551, 2017.

Livingston, G., Sommerland, A., Orgeta, V. et al, 'Dementia prevention, intervention, and care', *The Lancet* (390), pp.2673–2734, 2017.

NHS, One You, www.nhs.uk/oneyou/about-one-you/, 2017.

NHS Inform, Type II Diabetes: Causes, 2018.

NHS, Predictive genetic tests for cancer risk genes, www.nhs.uk/ conditions/predictive-genetic-tests-cancer/, 2018.

OECD, Alcohol Consumption, data available at: data.oecd.org/ healthrisk/alcohol-consumption.htm, 2017.

Office for National Statistics, Cancer survival in England – adults diagnosed, Table 5. Predicted estimates of one-year, five-year and ten-year net survival (%) with 95% confidence intervals (CI), for adults (aged 15 to 99 years) that would be diagnosed in 2016: England, 25 common cancers, by age and sex, 2017.

Office for National Statistics, Disability-Free Life Expectancy by Upper Tier Local Authority: England 2012 to 2014, Figure 1: Life expectancy (LE), disability-free life expectancy (DFLE) and proportion of life disability-free for males and females at birth in England, 2012 to 2014.

O'Keefe, A., Nazareth, I. and Peterson, I., 'Time trends in the prescription of statins for the primary prevention of cardiovascular disease in the United Kingdom: a cohort study using The Health Improvement Network primary care data', *Clinical Epidemiology 8*, pp. 123–132, 2016.

Park, D., Lodi-Smith, J., Drew, L. et al, 'The Impact of Sustained Engagement on Cognitive Function in Older Adults: The Synapse Project', *Psychological Science*, 25(1), pp. 103–112, 2014.

Prince, M., Knapp, M., Guerchet, M. et al, *Dementia UK*, produced by King's College London and the London School of Economics. Second Edition: London, 2014.

Public Health England, Diabetes prevalence estimates for local populations, dataset available at: www.gov.uk/government/publications/ diabetes-prevalence-estimates-for-local-populations, 2016.

Public Health England, Health matters: obesity and the food environment, www.gov.uk/government/publications/health-matters-obesity-and-the-food-environment/health-matters-obesity-and-the-food-environment--2, 2017.

Shahab, L., Goniewicz, M.L., Blount, B.C. et al, 'Nicotine, Carcinogen, and Toxin Exposure in Long-Term E-Cigarette and Nicotine Replacement Therapy Users: A Cross-sectional Study', *Annals of Internal Medicine*, 166 (6), 2017, pp. 390–400.

Sinclair, A., Ryan, B. and Hill, D., Sight loss in older people: The essential guide for general practice. London: Royal National Institute of Blind People, 2016.

Sugiyama, D., Nishimura, K., Tamaki, K., Tsuji, G., Nakazawa, T., Morinobu, A. and Kumagai, S., 'Impact of smoking as a risk factor for developing rheumatoid arthritis: a meta-analysis of observational studies', *Annals of the Rheumatic Diseases 69*, pp. 70–81, 2010.

Vernon, M., Ageing Well: What are NHS England doing about frailty? figures based on Kent Integrated Dataset modelling, aace.org.uk/wpcontent/uploads/2017/02/Martin-Vernon-NHS-England.pdf, 2017.

YouGov, Stiff upper lip may be preventing older people from sharing mental health concerns, yougov.co.uk/topics/health/articles-reports/2017/10/24/stiff-upper-lip-may-be-preventing-older-people-sha, 2017.

Chapter Seven: Where you'll live

Age UK, Age-Friendly Island, www.ageuk.org.uk/isleofwight/our-services/age-friendly-island, 2018.

Age UK Dudley, Get Cycling, www.ageuk.org.uk/dudley/activities-and-events/get-cycling, 2018.

Asher, L., Aresu, M., Falaschetti, E. and Mindell, J., 'Most older pedestrians are unable to cross the road in time: a cross-sectional study', *Age and Ageing*, 41(5), pp. 690–694, 2012.

Better Mobility, Charity Funding Options, 2018.

Department for Transport, Concessionary travel (BUS08) – Table BUS0821 – Number of older and disabled concessionary bus journeys (millions), 2017.

Department for Transport, Vehicles involved in reported road accidents, RAS20002, Drivers in reported accidents by gender, number injured, road user type and age, Great Britain, 2016.

GOV.UK, Renew your driving licence if you're 70 or over, information available at: www.gov.uk/renew-driving-licence-at-70, 2018.

Herefordshire Gov.UK, Refresher training for older drivers, www.herefordshire.gov.uk/info/200196/roads/191/driver_training/1, 2018.

IBM, Local Motors and IBM Pave the Way for the Future of Automobiles. Available at: www-01.ibm.com/common/ssi/cgi-bin/ssialias?htmlfid=WW112356USEN, 2016.

Ministry of Housing, Communities and Local Government, English Housing Survey, 2008–2017, New Households and Recent Movers, FA4121- Demographic characteristics of moving households

Motability, you can check your eligibility at: www.motability.co.uk/about-the-scheme/who-can-join/, 2018.

Newcastle City Council, Over-50s cycling school launched, www.newcastle.gov.uk/news-story/over-50s-cycling-school-launched, 2016.

NHS, Getting a wheelchair, scooter or walking aid, www.nhs.uk/conditions/social-care-and-support/mobility-equipment-wheelchairs-scooters/, 2018.

Office for National Statistics, Estimates of the population for the UK, England and Wales, Scotland and Northern Ireland, mid-2017, MYE1: Population estimates: Summary for the UK, mid-2017.

Office for National Statistics, Long-term international migration, age and sex, UK and England and Wales, Table 2.07, 2017-based.

Office for National Statistics, Number of British citizens resident in EU countries, by age group and sex, 2017, Table 1.

Prince, M., Knapp, M., Guerchet, M. et al, *Dementia UK*, produced by King's College London and the London School of Economics. Second Edition: London, 2014.

WHO, Age-Friendly World, extranet.who.int/agefriendlyworld/network/, 2018.

Chapter Eight: What your home should look like

Department for Communities and Local Government, A Decent Home: Definition and Guidance for Implementation, 2006.

Harrop, A, and Jopling, K., *One Voice: Shaping our Ageing Society*, Age Concern and Help the Aged, 2009.

Lloyd, J. 'Older Owners Research on the lives, aspirations and housing outcomes of older homeowners in the UK'. London: Strategic Society Centre, 2015.

Ministry of Housing, Communities and Local Government, English Housing Survey 2016/17, Table FA3101 (S418): Demographic and economic characteristics of social and privately renting households, 2016–17.

Ministry of Housing, Communities and Local Government, Dwelling condition and safety, Table DA3201: Decent Homes-Dwellings, 2016.

Ministry of Housing, Communities and Local Government, Overcoming the Barriers to Longer Tenancies in the Private Rented Sector, 2018.

PWC, UK Economic Outlook, www.pwc.co.uk/assets/pdf/ukeo/ukeo-july-2016-housing-market-outlook.pdf, 2016.

Scanlon, K., 'Private Renting in Other Countries', in K. Scanlon and B. Kochan, *Towards a Sustainable Private Rented Sector: The Lessons from Other Countries*. LSE: London, 2011, pp. 15–44.

Westerheide, P., 'The Private Rented Sector in Germany', in K. Scanlon and B. Kochan, *Towards a Sustainable Private Rented Sector: The Lessons from Other Countries*. LSE: London, 2011, pp. 45–59.

Chapter Nine: Friends, family and other folk

Argos Pet Insurance, Do You Treat Your Pet Like a Child?, survey results available at: www.argospetinsurance.co.uk/we-talk-pet/do-you-treat-your-pet-like-a-child/, 2014.

Cacioppo, J., quoted by Olga Khazan, 'How Loneliness Begets Loneliness', *The Atlantic*, www.theatlantic.com/health/ archive/2017/04/how-loneliness-begets-loneliness/521841/, 2017.

Co-Op Funeralcare, Our 2016 Funeral Music Charts, www.co-operativefuneralcare.co.uk/funeral-music-chart/, 2016.

Eaton-Terry, L., 'A False Dawn: Funeral costs rise again after a one-year respite', The Royal London National Funeral Cost Index Report 2017.

NHS, Advance Decision (Living Will), 2017.

Office for National Statistics, Marriage and divorce on the rise at 65 and over, data available at: www.ons.gov.uk/ peoplepopulationandcommunity/birthsdeathsandmarriages/ marriagecohabitationandcivilpartnerships/articles/ marriageanddivorceontheriseat65andover/2017-07-18, 2017.

Office for National Statistics, 2011 Census data, available via NOMIS table QS301UK – Provision of unpaid care.

Pikhartova, J., Bowling, A. and Victor, C., 'Does owning a pet protect older people against loneliness?', BMC Geriatrics, 14 (106), available at: bmcgeriatr.biomedcentral.com/track/pdf/10.1186/1471-2318-14-106, 2014.

The Silver Line, News, www.thesilverline.org.uk/wp-content/ uploads/2018/04/Loneliness-Isnt-Just-For-Christmas.pdf, 2018.

Spencer, N. and Weldin, H., 'Post-religious Britain? The faith of the faithless'. London: Theos, 2009.

INDEX